No Guts,
No Glory

No Guts, No Glory

Gut Solution—The Core of Your Total Wellness

Steven Lamm, M.D., and Sidney Stevens

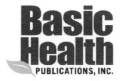

Basic Health PUBLICATIONS, INC.

The ideas, recipes, procedures, and suggestions contained in this book are not intended as a substitute for consulting with your physician. We are told that all matters regarding health require medical supervision. Neither the author nor the publisher shall be liable or responsible for any loss, injury, or damage allegedly arising from any information or suggestion in this book. The opinions expressed in this book represent the personal views of the author and you should check with your physician, medical professional, nutritionist, or naturopath before changing your diet. The recipes and information are for educational purposes only and the author assumes no responsibility for any adverse reactions to the information or recipes contained in this book.

Basic Health Publications, Inc.
28812 Top of the World Drive
Laguna Beach, CA 92651
949-715-7327 • www.basichealthpub.com

Library of Congress Cataloging-in-Publication Data is available from the Library of Congress.

Editor: Cheryl Hirsch
Typesetting/Book design: Gary A. Rosenberg
Cover design: Bob Jankowski

Printed in the United States of America

10   9   8   7   6   5   4   3   2

Contents

PART ONE

Your Amazing Gut . . . and What Can Go Wrong

1

Straight from the Gut

Life is not merely to be alive, but to be well.
—Marcus Valerius Martial (c. 40–104 A.D.)

Let me share a secret with you—and a guarantee. The biggest factor in determining your overall health involves an organ system that most of us ignore and even disrespect on a daily basis. This system is involved in a breathtaking number of important bodily functions that would probably amaze you. It's a surrogate brain, it helps regulate your metabolism and weight, it oversees most of your immune-system defenses, and it's the future site for new therapies and technologies that will enhance wellness and treat diseases that plague so many of us. Harm it, and you risk harming the health of your entire body. Pay attention to it, though, and I guarantee you better health.

What is this astonishing system that does so much but commands so little respect? It's your gut. That's right. It's simply impossible to be well if your gut isn't working right. Yet few us—even the most health savvy among us—really appreciate or understand what the gut does (which is far more than mere digestion). Nor do most of us care for our guts, as we should. In fact, many of us may be doing this amazing organ system great harm without even realizing it.

"But I'm not sick," you may be thinking. "I must be doing something right." And it would certainly seem that way, at least on the

3

surface. Yet, the fact is, many of the physical and mental disorders that afflict millions of Americans—including gastrointestinal illnesses and even some like autism and heart disease that seem entirely unrelated—begin quietly under the radar with trouble in the gut. Few of us are even aware of problems brewing until something really starts to go wrong. In other words, long after the difficulty begins.

Which brings me to my guarantee. If you start taking care of your gut right now—and I'm going to show you how in the following chapters—you'll not only avoid or reverse many debilitating and life-threatening conditions, but you'll also achieve your full vitality and vibrancy. In other words, you'll enjoy true wellness. Guaranteed.

MYSTERIOUS AND MISUNDERSTOOD

Almost daily at least one patient comes into my office complaining of a "stomachache."

"Point to where it hurts," I say.

Most of the time, they indicate their navel area or somewhere around their waist.

"Actually, your stomach is higher up, behind your ribs," I explain. "If the pain was there, I'd probably begin investigating whether you have a stomach ulcer. But where you're pointing is actually in your abdomen. That entire region—from your ribs down to your pubic bone—contains a lot of other organs and body systems, including your liver, intestines, gallbladder, and pancreas. What you've got is abdominal pain, not a stomachache."

About this time, most patients begin to look surprised. "I didn't know all that," they usually confess. It always amazes me how few patients really know much about this area of their body. Sure, they're aware they have a liver, and that if they drink excessively they can harm it. They know they have a gallbladder, but 90 percent of them can't describe where these organs reside or what functions they perform. In all honesty, can you?

I have a confession, too. It's not just patients who are in the dark about this complicated abdominal area. For many years, these organs confounded doctors, too. We have a better understanding now, but even the best physician is still occasionally mystified by the gut's complexity. When I began practicing medicine, I always dreaded when patients came in uttering that one word: stomachache. With so many organs there and so many things that can cause distress, it was—and still often is—a tricky call to figure out what's wrong, even with the help of CAT scans and MRIs. Abdominal pain can literally result from dozens of conditions—some of them originating completely outside the gut. I'll admit I've been baffled more than a few times.

Several Cases in Point

Not long ago, a sixty-two-year-old corporate CEO, who was in New York on business, came to see me. He was scheduled to fly out that afternoon, but for the last several days he'd suffered from abdominal pain that seemed to be getting worse. Finally, he called his doctor back home and was referred to me. Now, my job as a physician is to decide whether a patient's symptoms are severe enough to warrant immediate hospitalization or whether they indicate something less severe that can be treated in my office. In this case, the patient looked well and was in excellent health, but the tenderness, which spread over a large area of his abdomen, worried me. I sent him right away for a CAT scan, which revealed inflammation of his colon and appendix (a small tube attached to the colon that may be an unneeded digestive organ left over from earlier humans). My initial hunch that this was serious turned out to be right: he had acute appendicitis. We admitted him to the hospital that afternoon, put him on intravenous antibiotics, and operated in the morning to remove his appendix. He recovered quickly after that.

About the same time, another patient visited me, again for abdominal pain. His symptoms included bloating and diarrhea that had occurred on and off for several days. Now, suddenly, it was intensifying.

"Have you been traveling lately?" I asked.

"No," he said, shaking his head.

"Any recent illnesses or new medication you're taking?"

"None that come to mind," he said, then paused. "Actually, about ten days ago I did have a tooth abscess and my doctor put me on an antibiotic. But that wouldn't cause all these symptoms, would it?"

"Well, it certainly could," I said. And in this case, that's precisely what had happened. The patient's doctor had given him Cleocin, a powerful antibiotic that helped clear up his abscess immediately. However, as with even the best smart bombs, there was some collateral damage. The Cleocin (like all antibiotics) had disrupted the ecosystem of beneficial microorganisms inside my patient's gut that aid digestion, protect against toxins, and enhance the immune system. (We'll be learning more about the gut-harming impact of antibiotics in Chapter 4.) The damage was so bad, in fact, that it allowed a toxin-producing bacterium called *Clostridium difficile*—or *C. difficile*, for short—to flourish in his system. The toxin it releases often causes severe, almost intractable, diarrhea. Fortunately, we were able to clear it up by giving him a different combination of antibiotics to stop the growth of *C. difficile* and repopulating his gut with good bacteria using probiotic supplements. On the downside, though, he may be more susceptible to a recurrence of *C. difficile* in the future and will need to be cautious about using antibiotics.

More recently, yet another patient visited me for an abdominal complaint. In his case, the pain was more severe on one side of his lower abdomen and extended around to his back. He also had blood in his urine and kept vomiting. I had him undergo a CAT scan and soon found the source of the problem: a kidney stone, which he was able to pass fairly quickly once we put him on a painkiller and gave him plenty of fluids to drink.

And there you have it in a nutshell: three cases of abdominal distress, three entirely different reasons. In the first case, the problem was with a minor gut player and not one of the major organs that normally come to mind when we think about abdominal pain, like the colon or the stomach. In the second case, it was actually a tooth infection—completely unrelated to the gut—that led to this patient's abdominal discomfort. And in the third example, the source of the problem was an organ that isn't even part of the gut system, but rather is one that belongs to the urinary tract. In my thirty-year career as a doctor, I've seen gut pain result from a surprising array of conditions—everything from shingles and pancreatitis to a ruptured abdominal aorta and even a heart attack. You can see why it gets confusing.

THE AMAZING GUT

Even with our explosion of knowledge about the gut in the last thirty years, many doctors still don't fully grasp the influence this remarkably intricate, multitasking organ system has on our overall health. Not only are they perplexed by the multitude of symptoms that can originate in the gut, but they also don't take it into consideration when treating disorders that seem to lie outside its realm. It remains overlooked, both as the source of many diseases and as a pathway to potential cures. Doctors don't even really have the language to capture its significance and reach within the body. Older terms like "digestive system" or "gastrointestinal tract" just don't do it justice. The gut is far, far more than a simple digestion factory. Its organs provide a much wider array of services than simply grinding down the sautéed chicken breast you had for dinner and discarding what can't be used as waste.

The Hub of Your Health

The gut is actually command central for several key functions. This beautifully orchestrated system takes that chicken breast, breaks it down via a remarkable process, extracts dozens of usable nutrients, disperses them to every cell and organ system in your body to keep them functioning optimally, and finally excretes what isn't needed (itself a fascinating process). It also defends against toxins and out-side intruders, distributes medications you take to areas where they're needed, helps keep you at your best weight, and even carries on a running dialogue with your brain, regulating your sleep, your sex drive, and your moods. So important is the gut, in fact, that it could one day become a secret weapon for creating new therapies against disease.

Unfortunately, most of us, like our doctors, don't spend enough time thinking about our guts. Patients come to me every day, asking "How can I keep my heart healthy?" or "What's the best kind of exercise for losing weight?" They're worried about Alzheimer's, cancer, high blood pressure, and other big-name maladies. Sure, plenty walk in with abdominal complaints, but what they usually want is relief from the distress and a cure for what ails them. Rarely are they concerned about preserving and enhancing the health of their gut. Nor do most fathom their responsibility for keeping it in shape.

By the same token, few of us, including many doctors, really grasp the myriad ways we may be compromising our health by neglecting and abusing our guts. Throw off its ability to perform any of its key tasks or damage one or more of its organs, and you begin a domino effect of breakdowns that can adversely affect everything from your metabolism and immune system to your sexual, mental, and cardio-vascular health. Trouble in the gut has been linked not only to com-mon gastrointestinal maladies that grab headlines, like stomach ulcers, acid reflux, and inflammatory bowel disease, but also to seem-ingly unrelated conditions, like obesity, arthritis, cancer, vaginitis, and even mental conditions including depression, attention-deficit hyper-activity disorder (ADHD), and bipolar disorder. And new conditions linked to gut dysfunction are being uncovered all the time. For instance, recent research suggests that the gut may play a large role in forming our bones, and could even be key in the treatment of osteoporosis. The point is that ignoring your gut may actually lead to some of those frightening, big-name maladies you were hoping to prevent. Not only that, but as you'll see in the next chapter, you may be passing on health problems to future generations of your family based on what you feed your gut—or fail to feed it.

"Wow, I had no idea," patients usually say after I explain all this. I love to wow my patients! Frankly, it's one of my favorite parts of being a doctor—snagging someone's attention, educating them about their bodies, and arming them with information they can use to boost their health and well-being.

"That's why I like the word 'gut,'" I tell them. "There just isn't a better word for everything this system does. The word gut is part of our language. Think about phrases such as 'Trust your gut' or 'That was a gutsy call.' There's a lot of meaning in those expressions—they show the gut's place as one of the body's main centers of operation."

"Wow, I never thought about it like that," patients often respond.

"Most people don't . . . but if they did it could change their lives," I explain. "You just won't ever enjoy full health if your gut isn't working fully. So much of how you feel and how well your body functions begins in this core system."

UNSEEN ABUSE

Maybe you're like a lot of my patients. You work at maintaining a healthy weight. You eat fruits, vegetables, and whole grains as much as possible; take vitamin supplements; don't smoke; drink moderately or not at all; and try to stay in shape by hitting the gym, taking Pilates classes, or swimming a few days a week. You feel as though you're in control of your health.

If so, that's wonderful. But it is simply not enough if you want to really be well. You can't ignore the hub of health: your gut. It has to figure prominently in your overall health plan. And you certainly can't cause it harm. Yet that's what most of us are doing simply by being alive in the modern world.

Everyday Assaults

For one thing, we don't consistently eat the right kinds of foods—even those of us who try hard. For most of pre-modern history, the human gut was perfectly adapted to the fresh fruits, greens, and wild game our ancestors ate in abundance. However, in recent times, that sort of naturally balanced diet has fallen by the wayside in favor of factory-produced potato chips, microwave dinners, soft drinks, and other processed concoctions—foods pumped full of fat, sugar, salt, and preservatives that allow us to store them longer and prepare them faster, but that offer us little in the way of nutrition. We're expecting our guts to adapt to these never-before-encountered foods literally overnight in evolutionary terms, but that's just not how evolution works. What we've embarked on is a dangerous experiment in eating that's destroying our marvelous gut ecosystems as surely as any factory smokestack pollutes our air.

Mark Twain said, "To eat is human, to digest, divine." Just because you eat something doesn't mean it will be digested. If you're not taking in all the nutrients you need because your food doesn't contain many or your gut is damaged and not able to extract and distribute what nutrients are there, it can tip your health into dysfunction. You may think that smoking is the prime cause of illness in the United States. But the meager nutritional content of our food is the real culprit behind our poor health.

We also eat too fast and too much as we hurry through our busy days. It doesn't help either that our neighborhoods are teeming with fast-food outlets. Research shows that the more fast-food establishments there are where we live, the more junk food we eat. In other words, if they build them, we will come. One of the most unfortunate results of consuming all these high-calorie, low-quality foods is the rising obesity epidemic.

But that's not the only assault on our guts from the industrialized world. There are many more factors—things you probably never considered—that can harm this critical system. I'm talking about the harmful effects of continual stress and anxiety, which prompts your gut to release a hormone that tells your brain you need to eat more; yet another contributor to obesity.

I'm also talking about too little sleep, contaminants from the environment (like polychlorinated biphenyls and mercury), and the medicines your doctor prescribes—they all take their toll on your gut.

Frankly, no one should be surprised; the red flags are everywhere. Some 90 million Americans will see their doctors this year because of a "stomachache"—the result of constipation, irritable bowel syndrome, acid reflux, or any number of other conditions linked to improper care of the gut. That's more than will suffer from cancer and cardiovascular disease combined. In fact, the only thing more common than gut distress is the common cold.

Doctors usually throw pharmaceutical drugs at these gut problems—powerful drugs that often simply cover up the symptoms rather than cure the conditions, and that may make matters worse or produce dangerous side effects in the process. Then there are the millions of people who endure their gut ailments in silence, throwing over-the-counter medications at their problems in an effort to get relief and make them disappear. The result is pretty much the same.

But that's not even the whole story. As I mentioned before, the gut has its fingers in many other body systems. All these gut disorders that afflict so many of us can signal the presence of other problems simmering elsewhere in our bodies.

THE GUT SOLUTION

So what can you do? Remember in the beginning of the chapter I mentioned a secret—that a major key to health resides in your gut? Well, it's time to blow the lid off that secret. The truth is that you're really in control of what goes into your stomach and intestines. Food doesn't just find its way inside you on its own. Nor are you at the mercy of a stressful world or every toxic substance in it. In other words, there's plenty you can do to guard your gut against damage and enhance its ability to function properly—benefits that will extend to your entire body. And it's because you're in control that you have a responsibility to take better care of yourself. I plan to show you how.

No Guts, No Glory is not about procedures and medications—including ones from your drugstore—that can relieve your "stomachaches." As I said, most are really only Band-Aids, not true solutions that address underlying problems. Nor is this a diet book, although you may lose weight if you follow the advice. It's also not simply a primer on proper nutrition and better digestion, though those will certainly improve, too. It's really a total plan to stop undermining your gut and adopt healthier habits that boost not only your gut health, but also your overall health—and even prevent life-threatening illnesses and disease. It's about moving from intervention to prevention. It's about wellness.

Frankly, that's my main mission as a physician—to help my patients enhance and preserve their wellness. I don't simply want you to be free of illness. That's how the medical profession has long defined wellness. But just because you haven't been diagnosed with a disease doesn't mean you're well. In all honesty, you weren't well a week or even a month before your doctor diagnosed you with irritable bowel syndrome, or diabetes, or cancer. The seeds of those illnesses—the so-called lifestyle diseases—were planted years before they showed up. And when you're not well, it costs you, your family, and society as a whole, both financially and psychologically.

The good news is that many common diseases can be prevented with lifestyle changes, including better diet and exercise. In fact, some 80 percent of heart disease and type 2 diabetes cases and about 40 percent of cancer cases don't have to happen, according to the World Health Organization. In other words, the state of your health is largely in your own hands.

And that's what my plan is all about. I call it the Gut Solution—a simple step-by-step program that you can begin using right away, in consultation with your own doctor, to live a healthier, more vibrant life. Following it will not only remedy your "stomachaches," it could also save your life.

Embracing the Solution

In the chapters that follow, we'll take a look at this magnificent system—the gut—and how it works in tandem with every other part of your body. We'll explore the elegantly integrated ecosystem that each of us carries inside us, as complex and finely balanced as any watershed or mountain forest. So complex is this forgotten organ, it actually encompasses a surface area 200 times larger than your skin.

We'll journey through the abdominal organs, including the ones you're probably acquainted with, like the stomach, and ones that may be less familiar. We'll take an intimate peek at the kaleidoscope of functions each performs. I'll also introduce you to the many digestive enzymes and the trillions of beneficial microorganisms—including hundreds of species of bacteria—that call your gut home. In addition, I'll highlight the gut's remarkable array of roles within the body.

We'll explore how living in modern society can disrupt the gut's delicate balance—the product of millions of years of evolution—with often disastrous results. We'll look at the conditions behind our stomachaches, such as food intolerances, leaky gut syndrome, and dysbiosis (an overgrowth of bad gut bacteria), to name a few. We'll also examine some of the other problems that years of gut neglect and abuse can cause: fatty liver, asthma, diabetes, cancer, hypertension, and mental illness. I'll show you how to assess the health of your own gut, too, and accurately home in on what might be causing symptoms so you and your doctor can decide on the best treatment to get you back to full health.

Finally, we'll examine ways to reverse or avoid these problems and enhance the gut's ability to do its many jobs. *No Guts, No Glory* offers an easy-to-follow program that will empower you to take charge of your health. You'll find that much of the damage you inflict can be undone, and that it's never too late to begin. Certainly, the earlier you start following the Gut Solution, the better off you'll be. But you can make changes at any point in your life and reap the benefits. I'll show you how to bolster your gut, reinvigorate its digestive and immune capabilities to full capacity, and thereby boost your overall health.

A Three-Part Strategy

Using my easy three-part strategy, beginning with the Gut-Smart Eating Plan, I'll explain how to avoid processed, nutrient-deficient foods that are toxic to your body and replace them with natural, nutritious foods like raw vegetables and fruits, preferably locally and organically grown. Because they're richer in essential nutrients and contain a full stable of active digestive enzymes, they help your gut extract more nutrients rather than stand in its way. Additional dietary steps include:

- Eating plant foods with phytonutrients that offer special health benefits beyond what essential nutrients provide

- Adding more low-glycemic foods to your diet, such as whole grains, that aren't packed with high-glycemic, diabetes-producing carbohydrates

- Eliminating foods that trigger food allergies and food intolerances, which can send your gut into overdrive, hampering its efficiency and ability to function properly

- Taking time to enjoy and savor your food to promote digestion

Step two of the Gut Solution is Detoxification. The modern world hurls a growing mix of toxins and pollutants at us—almost more than our guts can handle. They're not just in the foods we eat, but also in the air we breathe, the water we drink, and even in the everyday household products we use. Just as eliminating toxic foods is one pillar of detoxification, I'll show how you can also purge your gut of environmental toxins by drinking more water, removing tobacco, alcohol, and other addictive substances from your life; by cutting stress, exercising, sleeping better; and by taking antioxidant supplements that aid your body's natural ability to excrete harmful substances.

Finally, I'll walk you through ways to Restore your gut to full function by supplementing with enzymes, probiotics, and prebiotics. Your body has a finite supply of digestive enzymes, and they diminish with age. You'll learn about the variety of enzyme supplements available and how they can easily replenish your gut's dwindling stores. I'll also explain how medications, such as antibiotics, decimate populations of beneficial microorganisms in your gut. Eliminating those medications is the first step, but there are also probiotic and prebiotic supplements that can help repopulate your gut's magnificent colonies of microflora.

The greatest part about the Gut Solution is that you'll begin noticing improvements in your digestion and elimination almost immediately. Just by choosing better foods, lowering stress and environmental disruptors, and boosting your gut's ability to function with supplements, you'll start feeling more vibrant, energetic, and sexy right away. You'll also find that you're sick less and have fewer allergies. You'll sleep better and feel calmer, too.

Granted, a healthy gut alone won't keep you well. Other systems in your body contribute to your overall health, too. And in the future, I may focus on these other pillars of wellness. But for now I want to shine a light on the gut—the center of so much vital activity—because it often gets lost in the shuffle, to our great detriment. You simply can't ignore this core component of your health without paying a very big price.

My hope is that you will have your own "Wow!" moment as you read *No Guts, No Glory*. I want you to appreciate the full glory of this marvelous system as much as I do and adopt strategies in your life that help nurture and strengthen it. The rewards will be many, and in areas you can't even imagine now. Treat your gut right, and it will treat you right in return. Guaranteed.

2

Your Own Personal Nutrition Factory

I am convinced digestion is the great secret of life.
—SYDNEY SMITH (1771–1845)

*M*aybe your idea of culinary heaven is herb-crusted Delmonico steak or arugula salad with goat cheese or even your grandmother's old-fashioned pecan pie. Perhaps you like an occasional glass of cabernet with dinner or live for fresh-squeezed orange juice with your morning granola. Whatever your preference, eating and drinking are two of life's great pleasures—social, relaxing, and satisfying.

If you're like most people, once you pop food into your mouth or take a drink, you rarely think about where it all goes or what happens from there. You just enjoy the experience. But consuming food and drink is only step one in an extraordinary process that converts all that delicious fare into the fuel your body needs to sustain itself and thrive. This is digestion, and it's the primary role of your gastrointestinal system—your gut.

TO DIGEST IS DIVINE

Even after thirty years of practicing medicine, I'm still amazed by all the gut does. It's a remarkably complex system of organs, blood vessels, hormones, nerves, digestive enzymes, and microorganisms; each

17

working at the right time and in the right way to carry out an astonishing array of functions. I like to think of it as a beautifully engi-
neered sports car; its finely tuned engine, cooling system, battery,
power steering, and electronic components all doing their part, alone
and in collaboration, to speed you down the highway in style.

As we saw in the last chapter, your gut not only nourishes and feeds
every cell in your body, but it's also the primary site for defending
against foreign invaders and toxins. (Your gut is actually responsible
for nearly three-quarters of your immune response.) It's intimately
connected to all your organs, and even talks back and forth with your
brain. In fact, many scientists consider it a kind of second brain. We'll
describe some of these extraordinary nondigestive functions and how
they contribute to your overall wellness in greater detail in later chapters. For now, though, I want to focus on the gut's main role: digestion (which itself is intimately linked to wellness).

As the body's nutrition factory, the digestive tract contains a crack-
erjack team of organs that work collaboratively, along with microorganisms, enzymes, and other components of the gut, to extract
nutrients from the foods and liquids you consume. Your gut breaks
down larger nutrient molecules into smaller ones that your body uses
for nourishment and energy, initiates their absorption into your
bloodstream for distribution, cleans out carcinogens and dangerous
substances, and excretes them along with other waste products that
can't be used or may be harmful. Everything in your body—from your
skin, muscles, and brain to your reproductive organs, eyes, and
lungs—relies on the gut to do its job so they can do theirs. Indeed,
your very life depends on your gut.

Gut 101

Maybe you learned about the digestive tract in high-school biology
class. There was the stomach and the intestines, and a few other now-
hazy organs. "Okay, it's been a while," you may be thinking. "I can't
remember everything, but so what? Digestion seems like a pretty sim-

ple process, right? Food in and waste out." Well, yes and no. On one level, your digestive tract is like a long, winding tube that starts at the mouth and ends at the anus. Food does indeed go in and waste comes out. But what happens along the way is what makes this system so incredible, and that part isn't simple at all.

Don't worry. I'm not going to overwhelm you with a textbook full of complicated digestion facts, though the topic could certainly fill a textbook. I do, however, hope to give you a sense for how beautifully constructed and complex this life-sustaining system is. I figure the more you understand about its brilliant design, the more you're likely to appreciate and care for it—and the healthier you'll be.

Your digestive system is made up of two types of organs: the hollow organs, which include the mouth, esophagus, stomach, small intestine, large intestine (or colon), rectum, and anus, and the solid organs (which most of us don't even realize are crucial members of the digestive team), including the liver, pancreas, and gallbladder.

Digestion works both mechanically and chemically, and begins well before you sit down at the dining table. When you haven't eaten in a while, a hormone called ghrelin is produced in the stomach, prompting you to feel hungry.

As you begin preparing a meal, the cooking aromas and your anticipation of how scrumptious it will taste prime your gut to begin secreting digestive juices so they're ready to go the minute you bite into something. In this case, let's say you're dining on a bean and cheese burrito. As that first bite of burrito slips into your mouth, your teeth mechanically grind the beans, tortilla, cheese, lettuce, and tomato salsa, while your saliva (a digestive enzyme) begins to chemically break down the starches into sugar. Saliva also lubricates the ground-up bits for easier swallowing and flow through the digestive tract. Once it leaves your mouth, each bite of burrito—now resembling something like wet mash—moves down your esophagus to a ring-like sphincter muscle that relaxes to let it pass into your stomach.

From here on, the digestive organs begin collaborating to propel your burrito from organ to organ, relying on gravity and wave-like contractions in their muscular walls. Nerves connected to the brain and spinal cord release chemicals that orchestrate this activity, urging organ walls to squeeze harder to push food through and later relax as digestion winds down. This action also spurs both the hollow and solid organs to secrete various digestive enzymes along the way to continue breaking down your burrito into macronutrients (proteins, fats, and carbohydrates) and micronutrients (vitamins and minerals).

Likewise, a vast network of nerves inside the organ walls reacts when it's stretched by food, triggering the release of even more digestive juices. At the same time, hormones produced in special cells in the stomach, small intestine, and pancreas begin flooding the bloodstream of the digestive system. They journey through the body's arteries, up to the heart, and loop back again, stimulating additional digestive enzymes and organ movement via a complex feedback process.

Here's a play-by-play of what happens as your burrito continues its migration through your gut:

1. **Stomach.** Once it enters your pouch-like stomach, powerful muscles begin contracting and twisting like a blender to churn the burrito mixture. Digestive juices secreted from the stomach lining are mixed in, including hydrochloric acid (prompted by a hormone called gastrin), as well as other enzymes that work to digest protein and fat. The hydrochloric acid has the additional role of killing harmful bacteria that may be lurking in food. Even more amazing, your stomach walls are actually protected from acid corrosion by a layer of mucus. By the time your burrito finishes sloshing around, it resembles liquefied soup. It's now ready to pass into the small intestine where most of the work of digestion actually takes place. (See Figure 1.)

2. **Small intestine.** The first nutrients to leave your stomach are carbohydrates and proteins. Fats, like any greasy substance, take a few hours longer to break down, and thus empty out more slowly.

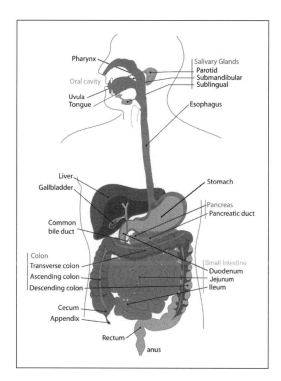

Figure 1.
The human digestive tract.
Reprinted from www.clker.com.

As the carbohydrates and proteins enter the first part of the small intestine, called the duodenum, nutrient breakdown revs up. Another hormone called secretin spurs the pancreas to send out a bicarbonate-rich juice to neutralize irritating stomach acids in the soupy burrito mix so that they don't harm your delicate intestinal lining. Special glands in the intestinal walls also release digestive enzymes; each one is dispatched on cue to further digest specific nutrients. As your now-unrecognizable burrito continues traveling through your small intestine, other players—the solid organs—come onto the field to do their part.

3. **Liver.** One of the main digestive roles of this marvelous multifunction organ is to produce bile, a yellowish-green substance that's stored in the gallbladder when not needed and squeezed out to further dissolve fat in the small intestine. The liver also helps ready the nutrients from your burrito for distribution to the rest

of your body. Here's how: Once these nutrients are converted into molecules small enough and in the right form for your cells to use, they begin to be absorbed through the walls of the small intestine via trillions of miniscule, finger-like protrusions called villi. As they cross over into your bloodstream, the enriched blood makes a stop at the liver first to be cleansed of toxins, medications, and other waste products before being ferried off for circulation throughout your body.

4. **Pancreas.** After bile from your liver has done its work on the fats from your burrito, the pancreas secretes enzymes that dissolve them even further. It also releases other enzymes that continue digesting carbohydrates and proteins. Then, as the nutrient-rich blood is finally absorbed through your small intestinal walls, the pancreas releases the hormone insulin into your bloodstream to help cells take in glucose for energy.

5. **Large intestine or colon.** What's left of your burrito once nutrients are carried off into your body (mainly toxins and other waste products) is next propelled into your colon. The breakdown and circulation of nutrients is mostly finished at this point, but important pieces of the process remain to be done. For one, water from the liquefied remains is extracted in the colon and supplied to the body to maintain proper water balance. If the leftover waste (stool) is too dry, the colon also adds water there for easier passage out of the body.

   Also in the colon, extraordinary colonies of beneficial bacteria thrive and act on the remains, furthering the digestive process. There are literally trillions of them (a few also reside in the stomach and small intestine), representing hundreds of species. In fact, the microbial makeup of your gut turns out to be similar to blood type: we all fall into three general gut types. So crucial is the role of these gut microflora, and so extraordinary is their ability to work symbiotically, that some people have even likened them to an actual organ. We'll explore this amazing gut ecosystem in greater detail in the next chapter, including how it protects us from outside bacteria and invaders and breaks down fats and toxins. But I do want to briefly emphasize here the importance of these bacterial civilizations in digestion.

For one thing, they metabolize food your digestive organs can't break down on their own, such as soluble fiber, which feeds the colon lining and keeps it healthy. Some gut bacteria also manufacture vitamins your body needs. In other words, these microorganisms aren't simply parasites living off your flesh and the bounty of your meals. They're active participants in the digestive process. In fact, they're essential to life.

6. **Rectum and anus.** Once your burrito has trekked through the colon, any leftover waste—parts that can't be used by your body, like the remaining fiber—makes its way to the rectum (the last few inches of the colon) where muscle contractions work to expel it through your anus as feces. By the time this happens, your burrito has made an incredible voyage of transformation, winding its way through twenty feet of digestive organs over one to four days.

ARE YOU HINDERING OR HELPING YOUR GUT?

The point of tracing the burrito's odyssey from your table to the toilet is to illustrate what an elegant system your gut is. The design is flawless; each part created to work with supreme precision and perfect synchronicity to convert the fruits, vegetables, dairy products, meats, and grains you munch on into microscopic molecules of life-giving carbohydrates, fats, proteins, vitamins, and minerals. Afterward, the harmful and unusable parts are discarded.

Normally, it's a seamless process. The gut works its magic without a hitch, and your body flourishes. You take it all for granted. However, when you start messing with your gut, things can go haywire.

Potential Problems

There are countless problems that may spring up along the digestive pathway. For example, you may have gastro-esophageal reflux disease (GERD) where the sphincter muscles that allow food to pass from your esophagus down into your stomach malfunction. As a result, stomach acid flows up into your esophagus, irritating and eventually scarring the lining. Ultimately, it can even block food from going down, making it difficult to eat at all. Or you may have gluten sensitivity and can't digest wheat. The result is cramps, gas, and diarrhea. You might have a stomach ulcer that leaves you in constant pain after meals, or a problem with your pancreas that blocks the release of digestive enzymes required to properly break down nutrients in your meals.

Whatever the trouble—whether you damage one or more of your digestive organs with medications, subtly injure the nerves or muscles inside your organ walls, snarl the regulation of hormones and digestive enzymes, or decimate your gut's microflora—when digestion isn't seamless, you diminish your gut's efficiency and your health suffers. Recall from the previous chapter that long list of maladies caused by breakdowns along the digestive route—everything from allergies, obesity, and cancer to autoimmune conditions, autism, and heart disease.

Why are gut problems so serious? It's because you rely on your gut to digest and deliver essential nutrients that your body needs but can't manufacture itself. You may be mostly focused on getting enough carbohydrates, proteins, and fats in your diet, but you simply won't survive if you don't also focus on taking in and absorbing the twenty-eight essential vitamins and minerals you need to stay alive. In other words, as beautiful as your gut's design is, it's only as good as the fuel you feed it. Put in bad fuel—meaning foods lacking in these indispensable nutrients—and your health will suffer. And so might your children's. One recent study found that the offspring of male mice fed a poor-quality low-protein diet were born with genetic changes in their liver cells that increased cholesterol production. The off-spring of mice fed a standard diet didn't show these changes (Carone, 2010). Bottom line: eating an unhealthy diet, even years before you have children, could put them at greater risk for later heart disease and other problems.

In fact, your body is *extremely* sensitive to nutrient deficiencies, even small ones. If you fail to feed it nutritious foods, you'll pay a serious price. Likewise, if there's a breakdown in how your gut metabolizes just one essential vitamin, the consequences are likely to be severe.

For example, vitamin B_{12} is normally released from protein with the aid of hydrochloric acid in the stomach. It then combines with a substance called intrinsic factor, also produced in the stomach, to promote later absorption in the small intestine. If something disrupts this process so you can't absorb B_{12}—if any leg of the journey goes awry or any organ fails to do its part—you'll develop a deficiency, leading ultimately to anemia, nerve damage, depression, and an array of other debilitating problems.

Along the same lines, if you have serious gastrointestinal diarrhea from an infection or toxin, you may not absorb enough potassium. Your muscles and even your heart will eventually give out. If you can't absorb iron in your food, you'll become severely anemic and could die. Without enough vitamin C, you'll get scurvy and your joints, skin, and heart will suffer. You can see how essential each nutrient is to your overall health and how crucial your gut is in making sure you get what you need.

Equally important is your gut's ability to eliminate waste and toxic substances (such as pesticides in your food) once everything is digested. As we just learned, both the liver and the colon are key members of the elimination team. When this system flounders, toxins build up in the body. For instance, you may have fatty liver disease (a buildup of fat in the liver cells) often caused by obesity, lack of exercise, and other factors. When your liver isn't fully functional, toxins aren't removed from your blood properly. Buildup of these substances can ultimately result in liver failure and a host of other diseases in the rest of your body. Likewise, when your colon can't remove waste properly because of constipation, and chemical-laden foods just sit, everything putrefies and toxins accumulate. These may damage the colon walls (even leading to cancer) or may be absorbed into the bloodstream, contributing to chronic conditions like fatigue, headaches, asthma, and many others.

Empowering Your Gut for Health

The good news is that none of these problems are inevitable. Think about it. Your gut interacts with the environment probably more than any other organ system. The only other two that come close are your skin and your lungs. Still, no matter who you are or how you live, these systems mostly face the same sorts of environmental exposures. They don't vary a lot from person to person. We all pretty much breathe the same air and maneuver through the same world. There are a few variations—some of us live in more polluted cities than others or reside near a beach, exposing our skin to more sun—but, all in all, we can't do much to control or change what our skin and lungs encounter.

The gut, though, is another story. In its role as provider of nourishment, waste handler, and the first line of defense against dangerous invaders, your gut is exposed to all manner of foods, pathogens, and cancer-causing agents that vary quite a lot between people. For one thing, we don't all eat the same things or take the same medications or use the same household products or practice the same lifestyle habits; there's a lot of variation from one person to the next. It sounds scary—such an important system at the mercy of a toxic world. But you actually have a lot of control over what your gut comes in contact with. In other words, you get to decide what goes into your mouth: chips, soda, and processed frozen dinners or fresh fruits, vegetables, and whole grains? You get to oversee how much you eat and whether you take medications that might upset your gut's inner workings. You dictate the amount of stress you experience and choose to either use or shun toxic household chemicals.

In fact, this is the very reason your gut plays such a critical role in your general wellness. Yes, it feeds your body, cleanses it, and regulates many critical functions. Yes, a lot can go wrong. But ultimately you're the boss. You can remove many of the obstacles that keep your gut from functioning optimally. You have the power to help it keep you well.

In the next chapter, we'll explore the amazing partnership between you and your gut's microflora and how nurturing this intimate relationship should be a key part of your healthy gut plan.

3

The Living World Inside You

Let's face it . . . the only position of long-term strength is interdependence: win/win.

—GREG ANDERSON,
THE 22 NON-NEGOTIABLE LAWS OF WELLNESS

*Y*ou probably worry about your weight, your cholesterol, your heart, cancer, and a whole host of other modern-day health maladies that dominate the news. You probably also wish there were more you could do to ward them off. My patients ask me all the time for some guarantee—a secret weapon they can use to keep themselves in tiptop health. Well, fortunately, I do have a secret weapon—and it just might surprise you. As we're about to learn in this chapter, one of the secrets to escaping these health robbers may literally lie with the trillions of bacteria, yeast, fungi, viruses, and other microbes that live in your gut.

If you could somehow shrink yourself and explore your gastrointestinal tract, as you would an uncharted continent or a distant planet, what might astonish you most are the vast populations of extraordinary life forms you'd encounter. I'm talking 100 trillion microorganisms—species upon species of alien-looking microbes of all shapes and sizes—that populate your gut. You only have about one-tenth that many cells in your whole body!

It's hard to fathom this teeming world of creatures and plant life that live unseen and unfelt inside you. Expand it to real-world scale and you'd likely have the makings of a mind-blowing science fiction film. "Okay," you might be thinking. "That's interesting and all, but enough already. It's kind of disgusting to think about—all those things swarming around in there."

Believe me, I understand. We've all been conditioned to think of bacteria and viruses as unclean and even dangerous. Our store shelves are filled with soaps and sprays that kill germs. It's nearly a national mantra—this obsession with creating a germ-free world. Except that some germs are good, including, as we'll soon see, the astounding societies of beneficial microflora that take up residence in your gut, assisting you in digestion, metabolizing fats, defending against toxic substances and harmful bacteria that enter your body in food and drink, helping you fight infections and disease, and aiding in the manufacture of essential nutrients. They even affect your moods, determine how well you fight infections and disease, and regulate how much you weigh (as we'll see in the next chapter). In fact, they're absolutely critical to maintaining your overall wellness.

It's an intimate, mutually beneficial relationship when it works right—an interdependent bond. They couldn't survive without the rich environment your gut provides, and you couldn't survive without them. However, when the wrong blend of flora and fauna flourishes in your gut, the health consequences can be devastating . . . and even deadly.

YOUR OWN PERSONAL ECOSYSTEM

The partnership between you and your microbial ecosystem begins at birth. As a baby makes its way down the birth canal and is delivered, fecal and vaginal bacteria from its mother quickly move into its colon (with a few also populating its stomach and small intestine) to help prepare it for life outside the womb. Before that, its insides are completely sterile. Interestingly, the guts of babies delivered via caesarian section are initially colonized in a more haphazard fashion, mostly by bacteria from the delivery room and hospital workers. In fact, caesarian babies may lack some crucial microbes, like the *Bifidobacterium* species, believed to help build the immune system in infancy. Vaginally delivered babies, by contrast, have an abundance of these organisms, and their gut communities are also well established much earlier, making them less susceptible to infections and allergies.

During the first weeks of life all that cuddling with family members and the milk infants drink add more microbes to the mix. Not surprisingly, perhaps, breast-fed babies have more beneficial bifidobacteria and lactobacilli in their guts than formula-fed infants, helping to guard them against an overgrowth of harmful microbes like *Escherichia coli* (*E. coli*) and streptococci.

By the time you're a toddler and eating solid foods, the composition of your gut microbiota looks something like that of an adult. From then on, you and these organisms live symbiotically, hopefully working cooperatively over your lifetime to keep each other alive.

Evolution of a Partnership

Just as your fingerprints are unique, scientists believe the makeup of your gut microorganisms is also unique to you. However, enough general similarities exist so that all humans appear to land in one of three main gut types—each one dominated by a particular bacterial species: *Bacteroides*, *Prevotella*, or *Ruminococcus*. Like blood type, your gut type has nothing to do with your age, nationality, weight, or gender.

There's a lot we still don't know about how and why these three gut types came about, and there may even turn out to be more than three, but understanding them could eventually help us further enhance our health. For instance, they might provide specific clues about how your body metabolizes vitamins, food, and medications. We know, for example, that if you're in the *Bacteroides* group, you have more bacteria that produce vitamins like C, B_2, and B_5. People in the *Prevotella* group have more vitamin B_1 and folic acid-producing bacteria. Knowing your dominant gut species (and which species aren't as active) could eventually help pinpoint your susceptibility to certain chronic diseases as well. You might be able to tailor your diet, lifestyle, and even medical treatments to take advantage of and strengthen your partnership with the particular microorganisms living inside you.

LIKE AN ORGAN

Their names are somewhat intimidating when you first hear them—*Lactobacillus casei, Enterococcus faecalis, Atopobium parvulum, Bacteroides fragilis, Roseburia intestinalis* . . . I could go on. But when you carry a healthy blend of these microbial species inside you, each one is a valuable member of your gut community, working separately and together to carry out a remarkable assortment of functions. In fact, these superabundant microbial colonies—hundreds of species in all weighing a total of two to four pounds—are not unlike an organ system. They are as critical as any organ in your body and as necessary as your heart, lungs, and brain. I can't stress this enough: you simply couldn't stay alive without them. Looked at another way, being human wouldn't be possible without these trillions of non-human companions.

Let's take a look at some major things they do. Again, my purpose isn't to deluge you with way more than you wanted to know (and believe me, there's a lot to know and more being discovered all the time). But I do hope you come away with a profound appreciation for these silent partners and helpmates that travel with you through life. Like me, I think you'll be wowed by the extent of their role in your body. Here are a few ways they keep you functioning:

- **Digestion.** As we learned in the previous chapter, your gastrointestinal system is a master digester. However, there are a few things it just can't break down by itself. Enter your gut flora and fauna.

These microbes produce enzymes that your own cells don't, allowing them to extract additional energy by fermenting food remains in the colon. The resulting short-chain fatty acids reduce inflammation in your colon, feed cells in its lining, help protect it from cancer, and help you absorb essential minerals, like calcium and iron. Gut bacteria also aid in the production of essential vitamins, like biotin, folate, and vitamin K, and promote their absorption into the rest of your body.

- **Metabolism of fats.** One digestive duty of particular interest is the role that gut microflora play in regulating how bile acids are metabolized in your liver. You'll recall from Chapter 2 that your liver produces bile (six kinds, in fact), which dissolve fats in the small intestine during digestion. Bile acids also make their way back to the liver where they help regulate cholesterol and other endocrine functions. Studies show that the types of microbes you house in your gut can not only change what kinds of bile acids go to work in your gastrointestinal tract, but may also transform their structure, altering their ability to emulsify fats. This, in turn, affects how much fat your body absorbs and stores. In one recent study, mice populated with a mix of "unfriendly" microbes had more LDL "bad" cholesterol in their livers (Martin, 2007). The types of bacteria housed in your gut may also affect how well cholesterol-lowering statin drugs work. A new study shows that people with higher levels of certain bile acids, produced by gut bacteria, had a significantly better response to the drug simvastatin than those with bacteria that produced other bile acids (Kaddurah-Daouk, 2011). Doctors may eventually be able to boost the effectiveness of statin drugs in all patients by using dietary interventions to encourage more of the intestinal microbes that create the helpful bile acids.

- **Metabolism of carcinogens.** Cooking meats, fish, and poultry using high-temperature methods, such as grilling over a flame and frying, creates cancer-causing substances called heterocyclic amines (HCAs) and polycyclic aromatic hydrocarbons (PAHs). In addition to their many other tasks, gut bacteria help metabolize these tumor-causing microparticles so they don't harm you. Your gastrointestinal partners also help metabolize other potentially deadly toxins, as well as fats (as we just saw), which when eaten in excess can actually raise your risk of many types of cancer.

- **Immune response.** Your gut is the body's primary contact point with the surrounding world. Everything you swallow—good and bad—arrives there first. Not surprisingly, then, the vast majority of your immune system resides in your gastrointestinal tract, and the bacteria that colonize it at birth and during infancy are crucial to its initial strong development. Afterward, they help keep it functioning optimally. One way is by lining your colon with healthy, thriving populations of gut microbes, creating an actual barrier against harmful microorganisms. Ne'er-do-wells simply don't have room to move in. Gut bacteria also communicate with your immune system, continually helping it to distinguish between good things your body needs and intruders that might be dangerous. In turn, your immune system can then create antibodies that attack invading pathogens.

A FRAGILE BALANCE

A healthy gut doesn't just contain good microorganisms. There are also a few villains dwelling there too. It's all about balance; as long as there are more beneficial microbes in the right proportion, their greater numbers keep the bad microbes in check—that is, they remain benign.

The ideal proportion is believed to be about 85 percent beneficial microorganisms to 15 percent harmful. When the populations are well balanced and stable, everything works in concert with beautiful interdependent precision. Your gut microbial network flourishes, and so do you.

But like any complex ecosystem, balance is often fragile and difficult to maintain. With trillions of microorganisms claiming your gut as home and relying on hospitable conditions inside you to stay alive, any number of events—from stress to antibiotics to diet—can tip the entire works on its side.

Think of your gut's ecosystem like a rainforest or an ocean. Rainforest trees provide habitat for wildlife, hold soil in place, absorb rainwater, and take in carbon dioxide while also releasing oxygen. Cutting down and burning these trees affects the immediate environment by wiping out local wildlife habitats, disrupting the food chain, and often leading to extinctions. This, in turn, affects people living nearby who rely on the forest for food and shelter. However, rainforest destruction extends well beyond its local impact. Destroying trees also contributes to climate change—a far-reaching effect that reverberates around the world.

Likewise, oil spills kill marine life, lay waste the habitats of surviving ocean dwellers, ravage beaches and marshlands, and decimate the livelihoods of people living and working in the area. But oil can also spread beyond local waters, affecting marine life in other parts of the ocean. Its damage may be felt far and wide for years to come.

The same goes for your personal ecosystem. Even subtle alterations in the balance of your gut microbes can unleash a series of malfunctions that not only reverberate throughout your gastrointestinal environment but also upset the larger environment of your entire body. Your health can suffer dramatically, and in ways you probably can't begin to imagine.

In the next chapter, we'll look at some of the things that can tip your microbial balance the wrong way and explore a few of the surprising conditions that may result—everything from obesity and autism to heart disease and cancer.

4

Dysbiosis: Your Ecosystem Behaving Badly

*The deviation of man from the state in which
he was originally placed by nature seems to have
proved to him a prolific source of diseases.*

—EDWARD JENNER (1749–1823)

*I*n an ideal world, you and the trillions of bacteria, fungi, and
other microorganisms living in your gut would be the picture of harmonious interdependence. Call it a win-win relationship.
They would get a perfect home and delicious, nutritious food. And
you, in turn, would receive the fruits of their labor—a variety of
crucial services that we explored in the last chapter, including manufacturing and helping you absorb essential nutrients, metabolizing
fats and toxins, and helping erect and maintain a razor-sharp immune
defense.

Like any flourishing ecosystem, though, things can disrupt the
harmony . . . and often quickly. When good microbes are attacked
or weakened for whatever reason, it opens the way for unchecked
growth of opportunistic microorganisms, much like the way invasive plant species might spread across a wildflower meadow if its
regular plant inhabitants are wiped out or weakened. The invaders
take over, often decimating the biodiversity needed for a healthy
ecosystem.

GUT DISRUPTORS

In your gut, this is called dysbiosis. It sounds bad, and it is. Since a healthy complement of gut organisms helps us stay well in so many key areas, any change in their types and numbers can lead to everything from poor digestion to fewer immune defenses. The result may be a startling array of chronic health conditions and even deadly diseases. Here are a few of the major disruptors that can topple the balance of your gut microflora:

- **Travel.** This isn't something most of us can avoid—or should. Nevertheless, exposure to new foods, different water, and unsanitary conditions in less developed countries is one of the most common ways certain nasty parasites get thrown our way—pathogens that our guts may never have encountered before. Most of us have had experience with Montezuma's revenge or whatever colorful name you apply to the explosive diarrhea that sometimes accompanies us on vacation. Even if you stay home, you may still find yourself encountering exotic bacteria in imported foods from the store or in restaurants. Today's global world makes it nearly impossible to evade bugs and other microorganisms that people once dodged due to geographic isolation.

- **Antibiotics.** It's ironic: we take antibiotics to kill bad, disease-causing bacteria. But good bacteria are typically wiped out, too, clearing the way for unfriendly species of gut bacteria to move in. So harmful are antibiotics that some research shows even one course of treatment can tip the balance of certain beneficial gut microbes for years afterwards. Even worse, the bad bacteria often develop antibiotic resistance in the process, making them particularly difficult to eradicate.

  Examples of how antibiotics impact gut microorganisms abound. Recall my patient in Chapter 1 who took a powerful antibiotic called Cleocin to clear up a tooth abscess, only to end up with an overgrowth of toxin-producing *C. difficile*. Incidentally, many hospitals are rethinking the blanket use of broad-spectrum antibiotics like Cleocin to help halt the spread of this on-the-rise bacterial terrorist.

Another common opportunist that often pops up after using antibiotics is the yeast-like fungus *Candida albicans*. An overgrowth can lead to yeast infections, fatigue, body aches, and gastrointestinal distress.

Yet another problem resulting from overzealous antibiotic use is the eradication of *Helicobacter pylori* (*H. pylori*) populations. It's true that infections with these bacteria can lead to stomach ulcers and gastric cancer. Certain strains of *H. pylori* may even bring on Parkinson's disease. As a result, doctors have taken to wiping them out with antibiotics. However, recent research suggests *H. pylori* has been part of the human gut for millennia, and plays an important beneficial role in regulating stomach acid levels, strengthening the immune system's ability to recognize and fight virulent intruders, and affecting the hormones that regulate appetite. In other words, keeping some in the mix, especially the right strains in the right proportions, may be a good idea. Wholesale annihilation of *H. pylori* with antibiotics does help prevent some problems like stomach cancer, but it also leaves you vulnerable to conditions like GERD, asthma, and obesity.

- **Poor diet.** Eating too many chemically processed, high-fat, high-sugar, low-fiber foods can also change the composition of your gut microbial and viral populations. Just think how a lack of dietary fiber alone might affect bacteria that rely on it to feed themselves—and you. Without it, they fail to thrive, and you don't benefit from their production of short-chain fatty acids, which help nourish and protect your body. And think about the impact of eating meat, poultry, and seafood from antibiotic-treated livestock and aquaculture. Just as taking antibiotics as medication alters your gut microbes, so does consuming antibiotic-laced foods, milk, and other dairy products. Consider also the toxic pesticides, fertilizers, and other synthetic chemicals you ingest at mealtime; all of them can disrupt the balance of healthy organisms living inside you. We'll explore these and other environmental contaminants in more detail in Chapter 6.

- **Stress.** There's no doubt most of us are stressed out—it's an unfortunate byproduct of our 24/7 world. Sadly, all that rushing and worrying appears to throw a monkey wrench in our gut microbial populations. In one new study, mice were subjected to daily stress by having to share a cage with an aggressive mouse. When compared to their non-stressed counterparts, the anxious mice showed a 20 to 25 percent drop in the proportion of beneficial microbial *Bacteroides* in their guts and a similar rise in harmful *Clostridium* bacteria (there are actually about 100 *Clostridium* species, including *C. difficile*). In other words, their gut organisms became less diverse with a greater number of unfriendly species. Not only did this impair their immune systems, but also their defenses were slower to recover after treatment to kill the *Clostridium* (Bailey, 2011). Not surprisingly, researchers have found that stress may play a role in gut disorders like irritable bowel syndrome (IBS), which causes cramping, diarrhea, and pain, and may even explain why it tends to flare up during stressful times (as do many conditions). My point here is that a poorly operating immune system—a key victim of stressed-out gut microflora—is never good news for your long-term health.

TALLYING THE DAMAGE

Just as we're dismantling our larger earth ecosystem through pollution, greenhouse gas emissions, and other destructive means, the problems I've just described are dismantling the balance in our gut ecosystems, perhaps permanently. Remember from the last chapter that the perfect ratio of beneficial to bad microbes should be about 85:15. Sadly, a majority of us are probably walking around with something closer to the opposite ratio. And the consequences of this imbalance aren't good.

The list of chronic diseases and ailments linked to dysbiosis is long and growing fast—in fact, it includes those very same modern afflictions you (and my patients) are probably most intent on escaping. Here are a few:

- **Asthma and allergies.** The Western world is obsessed with cleanliness. We use antibacterial soaps, live in airtight homes, pasteurize and process our foods, drink treated water, rely on antibiotics to fight infections, and use vaccines to prevent disease. It's called progress, but one theory—the hygiene hypothesis—suggests that babies and young children who don't exercise their immune systems by fighting infections on their own and don't move through a world crammed with animals, dirt, microbe-rich foods, and other germs (the way kids used to), don't sprout a diverse gut full of microorganisms. As a result, they fail to develop strong, high-functioning immune systems that respond accurately to outside substances. Lack of exposure to a broad array of microbial flora and fauna could be linked to the recent increase in allergies (an overreaction of the immune system to substances that aren't generally harmful) and asthma (chronic inflammation in the airways triggered in part by an overzealous response to allergens). Both of these conditions are indeed on the rise in developed, hygiene-obsessed countries.

- **Small intestinal bacterial overgrowth (SIBO).** A few microbes typically live in your small intestine (though nothing close to the number in your colon). Most of the bacterial arrivals there that aren't killed by acid in your stomach are blocked from getting into the rest of your body by the small intestine walls, and are instead swept out by muscle contractions for processing as waste in your colon. However, sometimes too many and the wrong kind of microorganisms get into your small intestine and stay. SIBO can occur for many different reasons. For example, if you take antacids, you may actually suppress stomach acid so much it doesn't kill bacteria before they reach your small intestine. Or food poisoning may unleash too many bacteria into your gastrointestinal tract for your small intestine to deal with. Research suggests that SIBO may be an underlying cause of IBS. It can also lead to poor nutrient absorption because the swarm of bacteria gobbles up digested food particles before they can be absorbed through your small intestinal walls.

- **Leaky gut syndrome.** Damage to the small intestinal lining can lead to inflammation that causes the walls to become more porous. One way this damage may occur is by SIBO. Remember that your small intestine normally blocks bad substances and intruders from being absorbed into your bloodstream with digested nutrients. Now, imagine hordes of bacteria bombarding your intestinal walls—too many to defend against—which eventually do it damage. In turn, this allows toxins, fungi, parasites, undigested foods, and other waste products that would normally be barricaded and passed out as waste to infiltrate the rest of your body.

  When toxins escape your gut, it kicks your immune system into action to fight the invaders. However, remember that having an unhealthy number of bad bacteria also weakens and scrambles your immune response. With leaky gut, your inflammatory immune defense continues in overdrive, protecting you even against things that normally wouldn't put it on alert. In other words, it overreacts—often with devastating effects. This may lead to several autoimmune conditions, including inflammatory bowel disease (discussed next), arthritis, chronic fatigue, asthma, allergies, type 1 diabetes, and even multiple sclerosis. Having a strong, diverse population of good gut microbes appears to both help prevent the inflammation that causes leaky gut and dampen an overactive autoimmune response.

- **Inflammatory bowel disease (IBD).** This group of intestinal autoimmune conditions includes ulcerative colitis and Crohn's disease. While they differ, IBD disorders involve chronic swelling and inflammation of the colon that can cause ongoing pain, bloody diarrhea, fever, and weight loss, and raise your risk of colon cancer. As we just saw, leaky gut syndrome is implicated in IBD, meaning that having a bad blend of gut microbiota is likely a factor. It's also interesting to note that stress (a major disruptor of gut microbes) seems to make IBD and other autoimmune disorders worse.

- **Obesity.** As we saw in the last chapter, gut bacteria play a role in how well your bile acids dissolve fats during digestion. There's additional evidence that gastrointestinal microflora affect how much you weigh, too. For example, studies show that eating a typical American diet high in fats and sugars results in an explosion of Firmicutes, one of the two main divisions of good bacteria in the gut, and fewer of Bacteroidetes, the other main type of beneficial bacteria. On the flip side, consuming a plant-based, low-fat diet reverses the proportions (Ley, 2006). This is interesting from a weight-gain perspective because Firmicutes extract more calories from food and store them as fat, while Bacteroidetes harvest fewer calories, resulting in less fat storage. It's not surprising then that people who are obese carry around more Firmicutes, while lean people house more Bacteriodetes. Interestingly, when someone loses weight, his or her microbial makeup shifts to look more like that of a lean person.

  Dysbiosis is also linked to low-level inflammation that promotes insulin resistance, which occurs when the hormone insulin loses its ability to usher glucose into cells and blood sugar rises. The result is weight gain and sometimes type 2 diabetes. In one experiment on rats, those given daily supplements of "good" lactic acid bacteria (*Lactobacillus plantarum*) had less low-level inflammation and stayed thinner on a high-calorie diet than rats that didn't receive supplements. Rats that were given inflammation-promoting *E. coli* bacteria (meaning they suffered from dysbiosis) gained significant weight when fed the same diet (Karlsson, 2011).

- **Type 1 diabetes.** This autoimmune disease occurs when your body mistakenly attacks beta cells in your pancreas, blocking them from producing insulin and allowing sugars to run rampant in your bloodstream instead of entering your cells. As we've seen, unbalanced gut bacteria and leaky gut syndrome may play a part in the development of type 1 diabetes, along with other autoimmune conditions. And conversely, proper exposure to a wide array of gut bacteria in childhood can possibly prevent it.

- **Heart disease.** For years we've heard that a high animal-fat diet, coupled with being genetically predisposed to atherosclerosis (clogged arteries), raises your risk of heart disease. Now it seems that how your gut microorganisms metabolize lecithin (a common fat in animal foods like eggs, liver, dairy products, fish, and shellfish) also plays an important role, and may even be a better predictor of cardiovascular trouble. One study of mice showed that having higher levels of three substances produced when lecithin is broken down—choline, trimethylamine N-oxide (TMAO), and betaine—resulted in more plaque formation in their arteries, a leading cause of strokes and heart attacks (Wang, 2011). Researchers don't yet know which gut microbes take part in breaking down lecithin, but we'll probably find that having the right kind—those that produce less of the three substances—offers protection against heart disease.

- **Neurological disorders.** Your brain and gut microbes "talk" to one another, and when the communication isn't working right because of dysbiosis, it may affect your brain chemistry, leading to behavior changes and neurological problems. Talk about a gut reaction. The trillions of microbes inside you play a significant part, along with your brain, in producing neurochemicals, like serotonin, that then circulate through your body. In other words, these microscopic helpers literally have the power to influence how you think and act. Indeed, scientific evidence increasingly shows that when populations of gut microbes aren't healthy or balanced in early childhood, they may send signals or cause changes that actually alter your brain structure for life—and not for the better.

For instance, strong evidence exists linking disrupted gut microorganisms to autism spectrum disorders (ASDs). One study found that kids with ASDs had a greater number of particular *Clostridium* species than normal kids (Parracho, 2005). These bacteria produce neurotoxins, which may have an adverse effect on brain development. Having a large cadre of unhealthy intestinal bacteria may also lie behind depression, anxiety, ADHD, bipolar disorder, schizophrenia, and many other mental health and developmental disorders.

- **Cancer.** We already saw how gut microflora help you metabolize cancer-causing substances that make their way into your body through food and other things you ingest. Since they also keep your immune system functioning optimally and provide your body with key health-enhancing nutrients—two things that affect your risk of developing cancer—it's safe to say their role is likely significant. In fact, research shows that certain gut bacteria, like *Bacteroides* and *Clostridium*, are connected to tumor growth, while *Lactobacillus* and *Bifidobacterium* have the opposite effect, blocking the formation of tumors. We already saw that inflammatory bowel disease (which is linked to dysbiosis) elevates your chances of getting colon cancer, but there's also evidence that altered gut populations may increase the risk of breast cancer, too. Additional research should connect more cancers to dysbiosis in the future.

HEALTHY RESPECT

This laundry list of what can go wrong between you and your gut partners probably sounds scary—and it should. The trillions of microbes that set up shop in your gastrointestinal system and accompany you through life aren't something to take lightly or disregard. The relationship between you is an intimate give-and-take, a dance of interdependence that touches nearly every function in your body. If you don't respect them or care for them properly, they won't take care of you either. In fact, they'll work against you.

Think of your gut ecosystem as a garden. You spend time doting on your plants and flowers, nurturing them, devising ways to help them thrive, and making sure weeds and other pests don't overtake and destroy what you've worked so hard to create. You should do the same for the hundreds of flora and fauna species in your gut.

How? By eating a healthy diet, lowering stress, ridding your cabinets of harmful household toxins, lowering your use of medications such as antibiotics, and supplementing regularly with probiotics and prebiotics. We'll learn more about these dietary aids in Chapter 10, but for now, let me just share a few points about their benefits. Probiotic foods and supplements contain live microorganisms—beneficial species like *Lactobacillus* and *Bifidobacterium* —that remain in your intestinal tract and help maintain an optimal balance. Prebiotics are made of ingredients that good bacteria like to eat and help them thrive. Research so far is very positive. Supplementing with beneficial bacteria or encouraging their growth has been shown to help with several health conditions, including viral diarrheas, allergies, ulcerative colitis, and Crohn's disease. Early research also shows probiotics and prebiotics may aid in fending off type 1 diabetes and obesity, and also enhance how well you metabolize nutrients and other substances during digestion.

The bottom line: the countless wondrous organisms at work in your gut are your partners in health. Keep them happy, and they'll return the favor in innumerable ways.

Next, we'll explore how evolution shaped our guts, and how poor food choices that go against nature affect its ability to function well. Obesity, food allergies, food intolerances, and fatty liver disease are just a few of the unfortunate results.

5

At War with Your Food

When diet is wrong, medicine is of no use.
When diet is correct, medicine is of no need.

—AYURVEDIC PROVERB

Our lives are not in the lap of the gods,
but in the lap of our cooks.

—LIN YUTANG (1895–1976)

Not long ago, a forty-year-old patient of mine came in for relief from some mosquito bites that were driving him crazy. He hadn't been to my office for nearly nine months, and I was surprised to see that he'd put on about thirty-five pounds since his last visit.

After discussing the mosquito bites, I finally found an opportunity to bring up his weight in a way I hoped wouldn't offend him.

"So, Dan, how are things going?" I asked. "Anything new to report?"

"Well, to tell you the truth, I'm a little more stressed than usual," he replied after a long pause. "My wife and I are having a baby, and work hasn't been as busy as I'd like. I'm really excited to be a dad, but I feel a little more pressure these days."

"Well, that's certainly understandable," I reassured him. "Hey, I also notice you've put on a little weight."

"Yeah, I've actually gained a lot of weight," he said, patting the extra padding around his middle. "It's been on my mind. I figured I'm just getting older or something."

"To tell you the truth, that's probably not it," I told him, "but I am pretty sure it has to do with the new baby and work."

"Really?" he said, sitting up and leaning forward.

"We'll deal with those mosquito bites, but let's address the weight issues, too," I suggested.

"Wow, that'd be great," Dan said, clearly relieved there was something he might do to stop packing on the pounds.

LOOKING FOR FOOD
IN ALL THE WRONG PLACES

Every single day in my practice I see people like Dan who've gained twenty or thirty pounds since the last time they were in, and it's usually a clue that something's up in their lives. About 99.9 percent of the time, with a little prodding, I discover that something has indeed happened in the last few months—and it's usually negative like a job loss, financial problem, or family crisis.

Chaos and periods of change almost always come with weight gain. I know it hardly seems fair. You're dealing with some big life event and suddenly you have to deal with extra pounds, too. But that's just how it is. The kinds of foods you eat and how your gut metabolizes them are a very accurate barometer of how you're doing emotionally.

Ideally, we should be eating foods for their nutritional value, not for their caloric value. We should be getting the most nutrient bang for our buck. Instead, though, many of us pick foods based on taste and use them like a drug for comfort against the stress and upheavals in our lives. In fact, new research shows that eating fatty "comfort" foods actually changes the signals between your brain and your gut, alleviating feelings of sadness (Van Oudenhove, 2011). In other words, fatty acids—nutrients in your in food—quite literally affect your emotions.

This might not be such a bad thing, except that comfort foods, which are usually brimming with lots of fat, sugar, and salt, harm your body and are actually addictive. In fact, many are so highly processed they don't contain much of anything digestible. We're not only hampering our guts and making them work overtime with poor-quality foods, but we're also starving ourselves of the nutrients we need for health. And in the process we're racking up the pounds. It's not surprising that two-thirds of Americans are either overweight or obese—our modern-day form of malnutrition. Potato chips, by the way, are the biggest culprits when it comes to that yearly weight gain that so many of us notice in middle age—bigger even than sugar-sweetened beverages (though they rank pretty high too, according to a recent study) (Mozaffarian, 2011).

It certainly doesn't help that junk food seems to be available wherever we turn. A lot of us end up eating far more of it than we should simply because of where we live. It seems we're not just a product of what we eat, but also of what's available.

Don't get me wrong. We all have a good bit of control over what and how much we eat. As the twentieth-century screenwriter Frank Howard Clark once said, "A child, like your stomach, doesn't need all you can afford to give it." But that's not the whole story when it comes to weight gain and weight loss—not by a long shot.

You may be surprised by this, but I'm not here to scold you for gaining weight. People aren't usually fat because they're stupid or lazy, or because they don't have willpower or don't realize that certain foods are fattening. In fact, there's a really amazing and complex interaction between the brain and the gut, which determines how much people eat at any point in their lives and what they eat. It's pretty tightly regulated, too, based on evolution. I try to reassure patients whenever I can that those extra pounds they may have gained are more a matter of hardwiring than a lack of discipline. And by understanding the process that led to their weight gain, they may be able to pay more attention to the signals ping-ponging back and forth between their bellies and their brains and reverse the cycle.

Here's a way of thinking about it. Our ancestors survived in times of stress and upheaval (which often meant famine) by storing extra pounds to help usher them through the crisis. This maximizing of calories is built into our genes. Stress actually triggers the release of ghrelin (the hunger hormone produced in your stomach), along with certain brain chemicals, to boost your cravings for carbs, sweets, and other comfort foods. At the same time, these hormones and chemicals slow your metabolism and reduce your ability to burn fat. This was an advantage during high-stress periods of scarcity. In essence, the gut-brain signals prompted people to search for whatever calorie-dense foods they could find and helped them store fat in their bodies more efficiently.

Incidentally, stress signals are also behind the inability of so many people to reverse this cycle and stop eating. Let's face it: twenty-first century life is stressful, and probably won't change any time soon. It mimics stress-filled times of famine or siege, so we're always on food alert. We don't go back to eating less after a "crisis" as our ancestors did, because the crisis never ends. This also explains why so many people regain weight after dieting. When you've been on tight calorie restriction, it feels like starvation or famine to your body, so the eat-more signals keep coming. Even the receptors in your mouth and small intestine that detect fat in food conspire against you. The more fatty foods you eat and the more weight you gain, the less sensitive they become, prompting you to eat even more fatty foods.

Is it any wonder, then, that chips and pizza make up about 30 percent of most Americans' diets, and up to 40 percent among certain socioeconomic groups, like Mexican Americans? I know it's probably not the best news if you're trying to stay trim, but bottom line: evolution favors weight gain, not weight loss. Our guts are still operating by the old rules but living in modern times so that all that comfort food meant to help us survive goes right to our waistlines and stays.

If you want to lose weight, yes, you have to start thinking in terms of eating foods for their nutrient value and avoiding high-calorie, low-quality choices. But you also have to recognize and calm those signals between your gut and your brain that may be telling you to seek out fattening, health-harming foods. You have to get back to feeding your gut the way it was meant to be fed. We'll be talking much more about adopting gut-promoting food choices and dining habits in Chapter 8.

ACCUMULATING FAT
IN ALL THE WRONG PLACES

One unfortunate victim of our raging obesity epidemic is the liver. Those extra calories we consume build up not just around our abdomens, but also in our liver cells, causing fatty liver disease, one of the biggest liver disorders in this country.

Your liver is an extremely crucial organ with an astounding list of roles that support nearly every organ and function in your body. In addition to its part in eliminating toxins (which we'll talk more about in the next chapter), it also helps metabolize carbohydrates, fats, and proteins. Plus, it's responsible for storing and distributing nutrients when they're needed, such as glucose (in the form of glycogen), vitamin A, vitamin B$_{12}$, vitamin D, iron, and copper.

Fat clogging your liver and subcutaneous fat around your abdomen often go hand in hand, and are linked to metabolic syndrome. This is a cluster of conditions that includes high blood pressure, elevated blood sugar, low levels of good HDL cholesterol, and high triglycerides (a type of fat that circulates in your blood). Having these together boosts your risk of heart disease and type 2 diabetes. If you're obese, you're naturally at higher risk for these conditions; but it's the location of your fat more than anything else that determines whether that risk is moderately high or off the charts. Studies show that if fat is around your middle and in your liver, your risk skyrockets.

Most of us know when fat is collecting around our midsections. We can see it. Doctors can even quantify it using an MRI machine. Interestingly, they can also quantify the amount of fat in our livers, using a machine called a magnetic resonance (MR) spectroscopy. But since few of us ever have this test done, we aren't aware that fat is simultaneously accumulating there, quietly degrading our liver function.

Maybe you've put on twenty or thirty pounds in the last few years, but you feel good. Your recent liver function test even came back normal. No sign of liver disease. But that doesn't mean there aren't fatty changes going on. Liver function tests only produce abnormal results when there's really something wrong—in other words, after you're already ill. But there's often a long stretch of slow decline in between perfect function and disease.

It's kind of like an air conditioner. It runs even when the filter is dirty, but not as effectively as it could. It's only when the filter is completely blocked that the compressor finally breaks down and your air conditioner stops working. It might seem as if it went kaput overnight. But it actually wasn't working well for a long time as the filter continued clogging up.

The same is true of your liver. If you're eating fatty foods, collecting subcutaneous fat around your middle, and your doctor tells you your triglycerides are rising, this is usually a sign that your liver isn't working in top form. The time to act is now—not *after* full-blown liver disease has set in. That's wellness advice you'll hear me give again and again in *No Guts, No Glory*, and it's the centerpiece of my Gut Solution plan, which we'll explore step-by-step in Part Two.

FOOD AS MEDICINE

It seems so obvious that food should be our medicine. We should all be picking foods with specific nutrients that help us stay well and reverse health problems. And our foods shouldn't share the same traits as our pharmaceutical drugs, which offer benefits but can also cause collateral damage in the form of severe unwanted side effects. Unfortunately, as we've seen, too many of us end up eating foods that do just that. They become our poison rather than our medicine.

One small example is fructose. Research shows that it can make fatty liver disease worse, actually causing scarring. This is because fructose (a form of sugar found in fruits, honey, and foods and sodas containing high-fructose corn syrup) is metabolized in a unique way almost entirely in the liver. This differs from other sugars that are metabolized more widely in the body. Too much fructose throws your liver into metabolism overdrive. Incidentally, high uric acid levels can be a tip-off that you're eating too much fructose. Uric acid is a chemical that's produced from the breakdown of substances in your diet called purines, and from too much fructose. Normally, it's also metabolized by the liver, but when your liver is already damaged from too much fat and is racing to handle all that extra fructose, it can't metabolize the excess uric acid fast enough. The result is a buildup of painful deposits in your joints—a condition called gout. Think about that next time you pop open a soft drink!

In recent years, more doctors have begun looking at food as medicine instead of always resorting to pharmaceuticals. This fascinating new world of "functional foods" (also called medical foods) is an exciting one. Many everyday foods are considered functional foods when they offer benefits beyond what's needed for basic nutrition. These include plant foods (like fresh fruits and vegetables, whole grains, beans and other legumes) and other unprocessed whole foods that are filled with disease-fighting substances called flavonoids or phytonutrients.

Functional foods also include pills and powders now widely available that are made from components of foods selected for their specific health benefits. For instance, in my practice I notice that a lot of my patients just can't find healthy foods all the time. How many of us really can? When treating those with metabolic syndrome and weight issues, I increasingly rely on medical foods, like UltraMeal Plus 360 from Metagenics (a powder filled with plant nutrients and soy or rice protein), which is tremendously helpful in improving their metabolic status. Another one I like is Mila from Lifemax. Made from chia seeds, this formula is filled with omega-3 fatty acids, phytonutrients, and many vitamins and minerals. It can be added to smoothies, salads, cereal, and other dishes for added nutrition.

There are also functional foods for depression, such as Deplin (a concentrated form of folic acid, a building block for pleasure-promoting neurotransmitters), and those such as UltraInflamX Plus 360 (also from Metagenics), which contain the amino acid L-glutamine and other nutrients to relieve inflammation caused by conditions like Crohn's disease. Researchers have even found that a powder made from compounds in the mukitake mushroom (*Panellus serotinus*) work to treat fatty liver disease in mice (Nagao, 2010). Another study recently found that an extract made from the mukitake mushroom actually prevented mice from developing fatty liver disease in the first place (Inafuku, 2011). We may see a product on the market for people one day soon.

This is an exciting new area, to be sure, and we'll be talking more about including functional foods and supplements in your diet, also in Part Two. What I want to emphasize here, though, is that before you can really take advantage of all they have to offer, your gut has to be in good working order. And sometimes gut problems lie with more than just having too much fat or fructose in your diet. They stem from your body's reaction to the food itself.

WHEN FOOD IS AN OBSTACLE

Remember the remarkable way your gut is able to break down food, extract essential vitamins and minerals it can't manufacture on its own, and help your body absorb them? Your digestive organs, enzymes, and the trillions of microorganisms in your colon all play a part, each carrying out its own tasks at specific times as food makes its way from your mouth to your anus.

We've talked about how the awful quality of our food is overwhelming and overtaxing our gut's ability to extract even the few nutrients it actually contains, leading to malnourishment and serious health problems. And in previous chapters we explored how troubles with your digestive organs and imbalances in your gut microflora can also block the absorption of nutrients—even if you're trying to eat right. But there are other ways you can fail to absorb key nutrients, too. Two of them—food allergies and food intolerances—are a growing problem for millions of people.

Food Allergies

It's hard to ignore a food allergy because you usually have an immediate reaction after eating what you're allergic to. The most common allergies are to cow's milk, eggs, peanuts, shellfish, wheat, soy, and a few other foods. Many allergic reactions are mild, and include hives, runny nose, diarrhea, and other gastrointestinal complaints. Extreme allergic reactions, though, can lead to a life-threatening drop in blood pressure and shortness of breath (known as anaphylaxis).

Food allergies cause your immune system to go into hyperdrive when it encounters a harmless food protein (allergen) that it identifies as an enemy. With most reactions, your body launches too much of an antibody called immunoglobulin E (IgE). In turn, that releases histamine, which initiates an inflammatory response to fight off the allergens.

Millions of Americans have food allergies, and they're on a dramatic upswing. As many as one in twelve kids in the United States are believed to have food allergies, and 40 percent of them have suffered severe reactions. One explanation is the hygiene hypothesis. As you'll recall from the last chapter, scientists theorize that in our clean-obsessed world, your immune system doesn't get enough exercise warding off real invaders and starts turning on benign substances that you encounter all the time, like food.

Whatever the reason for this epidemic, one thing's for sure: allergic reactions to food (as well as food intolerances) can cause inflammation in your gut that may contribute to leaky gut syndrome (which we discussed in the last chapter), blocking your ability to absorb nutrients properly. Interestingly, leaky gut can also *cause* food allergies by allowing undigested food substances to escape through your intestinal walls and whip your immune defenses into a frenzy. Afterward, every time you eat one of those "enemy" foods, your immune system springs into action. There's indeed a complex interplay of cause and effect that researchers are still trying to untangle.

The good news is that you can be tested to pinpoint the source of allergic reactions and eliminate those foods from your diet. Sometimes it takes a little more effort because the foods you're allergic to might be included as ingredients in processed foods—like eggs in a cake—without you being aware of it.

Another point of interest: some food allergies trigger other immune antibodies in addition to an IgE antibodies and some don't initiate an IgE response at all, making them both harder to diagnose. These include the following:

- **Eosinophilic esophagitis.** If you have other allergies and asthma, you may be more prone to this condition where, along with an IgE response, white blood cells from your immune system called eosinophils also build up in the lining of your esophagus in response to food allergens and cause it to swell. Remember, the esophagus is the passageway that moves food from your throat to your stomach. Items such as potatoes, peas, and shellfish appear to trigger this condition, which may include difficulty swallowing food, vomiting, and weight loss. The bottom line: if you can't get foods moving through your digestive tract, you can't get all the nutrients you need.

- **Celiac disease.** A protein called gluten, found in grains like wheat and barley, is the culprit here. Celiac disease was once thought to be a food intolerance (the result of a missing gluten-digesting enzyme). However, newer research suggests it may actually be an immune (allergic) response to gluten that your digestive enzymes can't properly break down. Instead, your immune system launches a non-IgE response, attacking the villi in the small intestine (remember those tiny finger-like folds in the lining that help nutrients get absorbed into the rest of your body). The resulting damage not only impairs your ability to effectively absorb many key nutrients, but also causes abdominal pain, appetite loss, and diarrhea (which in itself can also block absorption of nutrients because they pass out too quickly).

Celiac disease differs from regular food allergies, though, because its symptoms are chronic, and you may not know you have it unless your doctor tests you—meaning the damage continues day in and day out sometimes for years. Celiac sufferers often become malnourished, even if they're consuming healthy foods.

The only way to avoid symptoms is to eat a gluten-free diet. This sounds easy enough, but unfortunately it's not. Foods labeled "gluten free" often contain gluten anyway—possibly from being processed near gluten-containing grains. The Food and Drug Administration (FDA) is currently working on gluten-free labeling rules. In the meantime, it still makes sense to buy foods with the gluten-free label, but be aware it's not a 100 percent guarantee. Another little-known source of gluten are cosmetic products. Most don't specify that they contain gluten. It's yet one more way that celiac sufferers can inadvertently exacerbate their symptoms.

Food Intolerances

These conditions can lead to symptoms that are similar to food allergies, but they differ in important ways. Food intolerances don't marshal your immune forces against non-threatening food proteins. Rather, they're usually genetic, meaning that you're missing specific enzymes you need to break down certain foods or that there's a malfunction in the nutrient absorption process. Another difference is that symptoms often come on more slowly and are less severe. For instance, you're not likely to die from an anaphylactic reaction. Thus, you may ignore food intolerances longer than you might a food allergy. As a result, they may linger for years, blocking you from getting key nutrients and hurting your health. Common food intolerances include:

- **Lactose intolerance.** This widespread problem occurs when you can't properly digest lactose (a sugar in milk and other dairy products) because you're missing the enzyme lactase. Normally, lactase converts lactose into simple sugars (glucose and galactose) for absorption from your small intestine into your body. Without lactase, the unconverted lactose moves to your colon and is broken down instead by your gut bacteria, causing the sugars to ferment and symptoms such as bloating, abdominal cramps, and diarrhea to occur. The decline of lactase actually starts in childhood for a lot of us, about the time we're weaned. In fact, about 70 percent of the world's population is lactose intolerant.

  If you've got this condition, your instinct—or doctor's advice—may be to give up dairy products. But you have to be careful that you're getting enough calcium and other key nutrients that are readily available in milk. Many people find they can actually consume smaller amounts of dairy products without symptoms. Fermented milk products (like aged cheeses and yogurt) may also help boost your tolerance because the bacteria in them help digest lactose. Taking lactase enzyme supplements can build tolerance, as well.

- **Fructose malabsorption.** About 40 percent of us in Western countries have trouble absorbing fructose. The condition often coincides with irritable bowel syndrome (IBS). In this case, it's not an enzyme deficiency that's the problem, but rather a deficiency in the small intestine's ability to absorb fructose properly. In fact, most of us can only absorb a limited amount of fructose. When you consume too much—and many of us overindulge, as we just saw—the unabsorbed fructose moves instead to your colon where your gut bacteria are left to break it down. We end up with bloating, gas, and diarrhea (similar to what happens in lactose intolerance). If you suffer from fructose malabsorption, you may also fail to absorb key nutrients, including folic acid, zinc, and tryptophan (an amino acid that boosts serotonin levels in your brain, helping to regulate your moods). No surprise then that fructose malabsorption is often linked to depression.

- **Artificial food dye intolerance.** It's not accepted fact yet, but there's mounting evidence that foods like Froot Loops and Skittles, which contain petroleum-based dyes, may cause some kind of intolerance that leads to behavioral problems in kids, including ADHD. The FDA isn't quite ready to add a warning label to artificially colored foods, but it has recommended more studies.

MAXIMIZING YOUR NUTRITION

Many of you probably get it: you know that you need to eat more nutrient-dense foods and forgo the fattening processed stuff. You're all for nutritious meals that give your body more of what it needs. The trouble is, it's really tough to find fresh foods that aren't processed or laced with pesticides and other chemicals. You really have to go out of your way to get anything close to what our ancestors took for granted and ate in abundance. Even the most well meaning among us is likely to fall short at least some of the time.

Compounding this problem is that our digestive enzymes wane as we age. Remember that enzymes kick into action the minute you take a bite of food, with each organ secreting its own enzymes along the digestive route aimed at breaking down fats, carbohydrates, proteins, and other nutrients.

Unfortunately, we only produce a fixed amount of these enzymes throughout our lifetime. A case in point is lactase.

Leaky gut syndrome from food allergies and intolerances, as well as from environmental irritants and bacteria that inflame your intestinal walls, can also compromise your ability to release certain enzymes.

It all boils down to this: the fewer enzymes you have and the harder they have to work, the more gastrointestinal trouble you'll have in the form of gas, bloating, constipation, and other problems. And, when enzymes are missing or aren't doing their job of breaking down foods, key nutrients may fail to find their way into your body, resulting in vitamin-deficiency diseases.

It can pay to boost the efficiency of your digestive enzymes, and a good way to do this is by taking enzyme supplements. Certainly older people with declining enzyme levels can benefit. But so can people with food allergies, intolerances, and leaky gut. Because enzymes help digest foods more completely so they're absorbed instead of lingering in your gut undigested, they cut inflammation and other symptoms associated with these conditions. In fact, we all can probably benefit from taking enzyme supplements, particularly because few of us manage to eat nutrient-dense foods 100 percent of the time. We need help maximizing what we do eat. Many of us also have digestion issues we're not even aware of—enzyme deficiencies or small malfunctions that could be minimized with additional enzymes.

There are a variety of enzyme supplements available to help you replenish your body's dwindling supplies. For instance, there are broad-spectrum enzymes that can boost your general ability to digest everything you eat. Personally, I love Digest Gold from Enzymedica. There are also specific supplements that, say, help you digest gluten or lactose. We'll be talking much more about these useful digestive aids in Chapter 10.

In the next chapter, I want to take a closer look at some of the other things that can block full gut health—namely, our toxic world and harmful lifestyle choices. Just as toxic, nutrient-poor foods can keep us from optimal health, so can these poisons, especially when they're not properly eliminated from our bodies.

6

At War with the World

*It is no measure of health to be well adjusted
to a profoundly sick society.*

—KRISHNAMURTI (1895–1986)

*Y*ou're probably like a lot of my patients. You're not the picture of perfect health (who truly is?), but you're doing pretty well. No aches or complaints, good energy levels, no major gut upsets or diseases. You even got a thumbs-up from your doctor at your last checkup. Things are good, right? So why worry so much about your gut health when what you're doing obviously works just fine?

It's a good question and I have an answer for you. Your gut needs your attention because no matter how well you take care of yourself, the world bombards us all with things that may be quietly chipping away at our gut function—invisible toxins and poor lifestyle habits that don't often figure into our wellness equation, but that absolutely should if we want to achieve optimal health.

The fact is, modern life isn't that good for us. Not only are we presented with aisles and aisles of processed foods that clog up our gut mechanisms (as we saw in the last chapter), but these foods also often contain pesticides and other chemicals that cause us harm. What's more, we're assaulted daily with a stockpile of dangerous substances—

often through no fault of our own—that lurk in our cleaning and beauty products, in the air we breathe, and in the water we drink.

In 2001 alone, more than 6 billion pounds of chemical pollutants were released into the environment. Even low-level exposure to these toxins can do damage over time. Not only that, but the constant stress of 24/7 life also takes its toll and derails our ability to sleep well and exercise—and even drives some of us to use gut-harmers like alcohol and cigarettes. All in all, environmental toxins (some avoidable and some not) and our toxic lifestyle habits (which are mostly avoidable) literally overwhelm the gut's detoxification and elimination machinery.

I know you probably don't want more bad news about how hard it is to stay healthy these days—and this isn't meant to be a downer. Rather, I hope that by describing the lurking toxins that quietly degrade the health of your gut and the rest of your body, you'll begin to see how easy it is to actually cut a lot of your exposure. I hope you'll come to understand that improving gut health isn't just about better food choices, but it's also about lowering your toxic burden.

UNDER SEIGE

The purpose of *No Guts, No Glory* isn't to talk about every physical or psychological toxin that has an impact on your gut and other organ systems. There are simply too many to name, but there are some general categories of problem substances and unhealthy lifestyle patterns that affect most of us on a regular basis and contribute to our toxic load. As a result, our liver (the body's main detoxifying organ) and the rest of our cleanup crew have a harder time working at top capacity. Here are a few:

- **Chemicals, heavy metals, and other pollutants.** Go ahead. Take a guess. What do the following substances have in common?

  2,4-dichlorophenol   Monobenzyl phthalate

  Bisphenol A   Perfluorooctanoic acid

Butylparaben   Sulfur dioxide

Lead   Triclosan

Mercury

It's a scary-sounding list, and, sadly, these are just a few of the 219 harmful chemicals and heavy metals the Centers for Disease Control and Prevention has discovered so far in human urine and blood since it began testing for them in 1999—toxins that are found all around us in plastics, herbicides, non-stick cookware, tap water, vinyl flooring, cosmetics, antibacterial soaps, food additives and preservatives, and in the air (from industrial emissions). These harmful substances silently invade our bodies, and the results can be ruinous to our health when they're not properly excreted and remain inside us. Here are some of the main sources of chemicals and pollutants that contribute to our toxic body burdens:

o *Personal care products and cosmetics.* Store shelves are filled with thousands of beauty and hygiene aids that harbor many chemicals, including phthalates, a key component of plastics that can damage the liver, kidneys, and reproductive system. Everything from nail polish and perfume to lotion and hair spray contains these and other toxic chemicals, many of which don't have good safety data to support their use and often aren't even listed on product labels. That's because the Food and Drug Administration (FDA) has virtually no regulatory authority over beauty and cosmetic products, meaning manufacturers can put almost anything them.

o *Food additives, preservatives, and pesticides.* The food you eat every day also has chemicals in it—unless, of course, you buy only organically grown, fresh, unprocessed foods or grow your own without synthetic pesticides or fertilizers. Substances lurking in your food include additives to preserve it or enhance its flavor or color, pesticide residues, and antibiotics used to keep livestock or fish living in close quarters from getting sick. Unlike cosmetics, the FDA does regulate food additives, and food manufacturers must submit safety studies before they sell products in stores. But the FDA doesn't test food products itself to verify information provided by the manufacturers. Many additives, including Red Dye #40 and butylated hydroxytoluene (BHT), remain controversial because a few studies suggest they may be linked to health problems such as cancer. In fact, some additives, originally thought to be safe, have since been shown to be dangerous with additional research and are now banned. There is also controversy about the safety of the 1.3 million tons of pesticides used in the United States annually. They are regulated by the FDA, the Environmental Protection Agency (EPA), and the U.S. Department of Agriculture (USDA), but many pesticides were approved for use before studies were done linking them to severe health problems, such as cancer. What's more, the federal government doesn't monitor imported foods as closely, so pesticide levels may be high in foods coming from countries without strict pesticide regulations.

○ *Air pollution.* About half of all Americans live in areas where air levels of ozone and particulate matter (which can contain diesel soot, nitrates from fertilizers, sulfate aerosols, lead, and arsenic) are at extremely unhealthy levels, and many others live in places where air quality is at least somewhat unhealthy. Pollutants are emitted from vehicles, power plants, industrial sites, and other sources, entering our bodies through our lungs. Air pollution regulations have reduced the amounts of many airborne toxins, but not all, meaning most of us are likely breathing in harmful substances at least some of the time.

○ *Drinking water.* Pollutants end up in our water—and our bodies —from agricultural and industrial runoff, precipitation, and seepage of toxins into the groundwater. Over 300 hazardous pollutants have been found in tap water in recent years, directly affecting some 256 million Americans. Over half the chemicals discovered are not regulated (including the rocket fuel component perchlorate, the refrigerant Freon, the weed killer metolachlor, and the industrial solvent acetone). What's more, those that are regulated (such as arsenic and lead) often exceed legal limits.

- **Chronic stress.** Your gut is full of nerves and is in continual communication with your brain. In fact, your gut "brain" shares many of the same functions. When you're stressed, your brain sends out distress signals to your gut. Short-term anxiety isn't the problem. It's unrelenting stress that your gut—and the rest of your body—can't handle. And it leads to everything from an upset stomach and gastrointestinal disorders to lowered immune function, dysbiosis (a disruption of good gut bacteria that we discussed in Chapter 4), and even sexual dysfunction. Continual worry and upset also prompt food cravings, as we saw in the last chapter, that drive you to eat more than you should, particularly gut-harming high-fat, high-carb, processed comfort foods that may contain artificial dyes and preservatives. It becomes a destructive cycle: the more stressed you are, the more toxic foods, fat, and other harmful substances you put into your body. This, in turn, puts more stress on your liver (remember fatty liver disease) and other gut organs.

- **Alcohol, tobacco, and drugs.** Too much alcohol can affect nearly every part of the digestive tract, including interfering with gastric acid secretion in the stomach, promoting dysbiosis, hampering nutrient absorption, and harming the liver.

  Due to the many dangerous chemicals in tobacco that make their way to your gut, smokers are more likely to suffer from a litany of digestive disorders, such as gallstones, peptic ulcers, liver disease, Crohn's disease, and several types of gastrointestinal cancers. Smoking also impairs pancreatic duct cell function, even years after someone quits; so even former smokers are at risk for gut issues.

  Recreational drugs also do damage to your gut. Cocaine, for instance, constricts the blood vessels that supply your gastrointestinal system, limiting oxygen and leading to ulcers and other problems.

- **Medicines.** Many prescription and over-the-counter medications can also do your gut harm. For instance, nonsteroidal anti-inflammatory drugs (NSAIDs) may irritate the stomach lining and lead to ulcers. High blood pressure drugs and antacids (ironically, the very medicine people take to remedy their gastric discomfort) often cause gut issues as well, including constipation that halts the elimination of wastes. And, as we've seen, antibiotics can lead to dysbiosis, as can antacids that cut bacteria-killing stomach acid and allow an overgrowth of bad bacteria in the small intestine. Liver function may also be damaged by too much acetaminophen, steroids, and other medications—another ironic twist because one of the liver's main functions is to process medications that instead end up hurting it.

- **Sleep deprivation.** In a nasty trick, sleeplessness disrupts the very same hunger hormones that stress does, prompting all those cravings for unhealthy comfort foods we just discussed. In turn, the resulting weight gain and obesity not only fuels fatty liver disease, but also depression, which prompts a vicious cycle of more bingeing—and not just on food. You may also turn to gut-injuring alcohol and other addictive substances.

- **Lack of exercise.** Inactivity can slow blood flow to your gut organs, putting the kibosh on their ability to function fully. Couch potatoes also tend to suffer more from gallstones and constipation. And when you don't move much, neither do the toxins and other waste in your colon!

DEFENDING YOUR LIFE

Your gut is so critical to your body's defense network because everything entering your mouth makes its way there first—all the beneficial substances and all the detrimental ones, too. If you didn't have to contend with a crazy work schedule, chemical fertilizer residues on your vegetables, and hazardous chemicals in your deodorant on a daily basis, your gut's defense system would probably be able to handle everything just fine.

It's actually an amazing setup—kind of like a magnificently trained army, air force, and navy all in one, with your liver at the top of the command chain. When everything is in fighting shape, it's a seamless operation that works beautifully to keep you safe from the world's dangers. Your gut digests and helps distribute the good things your body needs to flourish, and detoxifies and eliminates the bad things that aren't needed or shouldn't be there. These include toxins we already discussed, as well as those manufactured during normal bodily functions (such as damaged cells and old hormones like estrogen and testosterone).

Defense starts as soon as food enters the acidic environment of your stomach. Any pathogens that survive, plus other toxic substances that the stomach can't neutralize, next pass into your small intestine where they bump up against the intestinal lining—one of your body's most intricate lines of defense. The walls of your small intestine are covered with immune cells that block and neutralize many health-harming substances and microorganisms, so they aren't absorbed into your bloodstream when digested nutrients are ready for distribution throughout your body. Instead, they can be discarded as waste.

Next stop: the liver—detoxifier extraordinaire. In addition to its many other critical duties, including maintaining hormone balance, creating proteins, and storing energy, vitamins, and minerals, your multitasking liver is also responsible for cleansing your blood of all toxins. Once nutrients cross into the bloodstream through the small intestinal walls, the enriched blood takes a swing through your liver where any remaining problem substances are cleaned out before the nutrient-laden blood departs to feed your cells.

The liver converts these toxins—most of which are fat soluble (meaning they dissolve in fat)—to harmless water-soluble chemicals, which are more easily eliminated from your body. Depending on what they are, they're sent either to the kidneys so they can be excreted in your urine or are mixed with bile and sent to the colon where they're passed out in your feces. I simply can't say enough about the liver's importance in helping rid your body of bad substances.

Unfortunately, your gut's detoxification machinery only functions well as long as the toxic load and poor lifestyle habits it's expected to handle don't get out of control. When there are too many dangers or your gut integrity is compromised for any reason, this finely tuned process may become too overwhelmed to properly detoxify and eliminate poisons or overcome poisonous habits.

For instance, too many toxins, pesticides, and medications may contribute to leaky gut syndrome by inflaming your intestinal lining and causing spaces to form between the cells. When these substances escape through the permeable walls, the deluge overwhelms your liver's ability to cleanse everything. And if your liver is already damaged itself from fatty liver disease or another problem, it's even less able to process the overload. The results can be catastrophic to your health.

For example, all those toxins that are supposed to be converted to water-soluble substances for excretion may instead make their way back to batter the small intestinal lining again, leaving it even more porous. They can also keep recirculating through your body and end up being stored in fat tissue, where they may damage cells and lead to a host of diseases, including cancer. Or they may make their way to your colon, where they might sit because of constipation caused by dehydration, a poor diet lacking in necessary fiber, inactivity, irritable bowel syndrome, or diverticulitis (small pouches that form in weakened areas of the colon walls and obstruct passage of waste). Bottom line: when waste doesn't make its way out of your colon in a timely fashion, it can languish for days, damaging the lining and even allowing toxins to be absorbed into your body again.

THE GUT SOLUTION

The good news is, you can make changes in your life to ease this toxic burden and help your gut help you. This is the second step of the Gut Solution—Detoxification. It means ridding your life of as much stress as possible, along with chemicals and pollutants that can be avoided with a little effort. It also means exercising more, sleeping better, and feeding your liver healthy nutrients and supplements that protect it from harm and enhance its detoxification abilities.

We'll be talking more about this and the other steps of my Gut Solution plan in Part Two. In addition to Detoxification, I'll take you through step one—the Gut-Smart Eating Plan—which emphasizes allowing time to develop a relationship with your food, forgoing highly processed, low-fiber, low-nutrition foods in exchange for more nutrient-dense foods, and avoiding foods that trigger food allergies and intolerances that can prevent you from absorbing essential nutrients.

We'll also discuss Restoring your gut's ability to do its job by supplementing with enzymes, probiotics, and prebiotics (step three). My aim in *No Guts, No Glory* is to help you incorporate these gut-changing strategies into your life as effortlessly as possible so you can enjoy optimal health right away.

Before we explore my three-part strategy, though, it may be helpful to first see how well your own gut is functioning. In the next chapter, we'll learn how to do a simple gut check to sniff out problem areas so you can customize the Gut Solution to your specific needs.

7

Gut Check

My soul is dark with stormy riot,
Directly traceable to diet.

—SAMUEL HOFFENSTEIN (1890–1947)

*I*magine yourself eating a portobello mushroom and swiss cheese sandwich on rye. You bite, chew, and swallow. Mushrooms, cheese, and bread make their way through your digestive tract as nutrients are extracted and waste is passed out.

If all goes well, you won't feel or notice a thing. The entire process will be seamless and effortless, much like breathing. Food in, waste out. Regular bowel movements. No constipation or diarrhea. No sleepiness, indigestion, or acid reflux. In fact, the only thing you should feel after eating is *not hungry*. But what if you notice bloating, gas, runny bowels, pain, or any other gastrointestinal symptom? How can you tell what's causing it? Should you call your doctor or wait? In other words, just how can you assess the state of your gut?

Actually, giving yourself a gut check is easier than you might think, and I'm going to show you how. Not only will it help you pinpoint problem areas that might call for a change of lifestyle, but it can also give your doctor more accurate information to make a quicker and better diagnosis if something more serious is going on.

GUT FEELINGS

Before you decide you don't need to do a gut check because you don't have any glaring gastrointestinal problems, just hear me out. Almost all of us have some kind of gut issue whether we know it or not, and here's why: it's nearly impossible to eat the kinds of foods our guts were made to digest 100 percent of the time. As a patient recently said to me, "It's easy not to eat too much, but it's difficult to find food that's good to eat."

Humans are constructed to consume fresh, raw fruits, succulent (non-starchy) vegetables, leafy greens, nuts, and seeds. That's it. No pizza, salami sandwiches, apple pie, or root beer. Your gut evolved over millions of years to perfectly handle what our caveman and cavewoman ancestors ate: nothing but unprocessed, uncooked, low-carb plant foods—the optimum human diet.

But how many of us eat this way all the time? Probably, not many. Sure, you may know someone who lives this kind of culinary lifestyle or comes close. But for the vast majority of us, it's virtually impossible to stick with a diet like this—and probably not much fun either. We live in the real world of grocery stores and restaurants, deadlines and meals on the run—not off the grid, growing our own organic vegetables and foraging for wild greens and seeds.

If you're one of the rare few who can pull off the optimum human diet, then congratulations! Your gut will thank you with years of good health. But for most of us—even those who try really hard to eat healthfully—mealtimes are likely to include at least a few foods that don't mesh with our gut's physiology. For instance, rice, beans, whole-grain breads, and potatoes are often touted as healthy. And, relatively speaking, they're better than a lot of other choices. In small amounts, your gut can handle legumes, grains, and starchy vegetables pretty well. But they're not ideal foods for full health. That's because they're relative newcomers in evolutionary terms; they only arrived on the scene within the last few thousand years when humans transitioned from being hunter/gatherers to farmers. Evolution is slow, and your gut simply hasn't caught up yet with this shift in diet and lifestyle.

Dairy products and oils (particularly good oils such as monounsaturates and polyunsaturates) also make the healthy list sometimes. But your gut is even less able to handle these foods. And forget about meat, eggs, and processed modern-age concoctions filled with refined starches, sugars, and artificial colors and flavors. These are simply incompatible with your digestive apparatus. And as long as you continue dining on foods that aren't compatible with your gut—whether slightly incompatible or really incompatible—there's going to be a price to pay.

Frankly, this is why millions of us see our doctor for gastrointestinal disorders, and why the same numbers are probably tolerating some level of gut discomfort in silence. It also explains why so many of us suffer from lifestyle diseases, like heart disease, cancer, Alzheimer's, autoimmune disorders, food allergies, depression, obesity, and a host of other maladies caused in large part by poor diet and health habits. After all, who doesn't consume eggs or meat or refined starches at least some of the time—and probably most of the time? Let's be honest, it's the standard American diet, and it's how a majority of us eat.

Okay, so I'm probably not going to convince you to embrace your inner caveperson and eat only fresh fruits, vegetables, seeds, nuts, and leafy greens. I probably can't even get you to completely give up the worst culprits. And that's okay. I'm a realist. A lot of those culprits do taste good . . . filet mignon, ice cream, kettle-cooked potato chips, and chocolate cake, to name just a few. I'm not here to take away your favorite treats. Indulging your taste buds once in a while is one of life's great pleasures, and your gut can certainly handle a few of these goodies. But that's the key: *a few*. Almost all of us can do better—and without too much effort either.

If I can convince you to eat healthier or make better selections 75 or 80 percent of the time, you'll be limiting a lot of the damage and boosting your health big time. If you start including more of those raw, fresh fruits and vegetables that your gut was made to digest; cutting down on the starchy vegetables, grains, and dairy products that aren't really well suited to your gut's anatomy; and eliminating most of the worst foods (what I like to call the three food groups: hamburgers, soda, and fries); then you'll avoid a lot of the gut complaints and health disorders that afflict so many of us. You may not avoid them all. As I said, nearly all of us have some degree of digestive trouble just by virtue of living in this century. But if you munch with your gut in mind most of the time, your problems are likely to be milder and more manageable than if you eat without regard for your digestive machinery.

THINK LIKE A DOCTOR

So if most of us have a gut issue or two, just how do you know what yours are? The first step is to pay attention. With most organ systems, like your heart or joints, pain is what usually catches your attention first. But your gut is different because pain is just one of the many symptoms that might show up. You could feel full, for instance, immediately after biting into a sandwich. You might have trouble swallowing or your stomach might be bloated and stay that way longer than usual. You might notice gas or constipation or diarrhea or a host of other changes in your bowels. Anything that draws your attention to your gut is its way of telling you something's not working properly.

There are many useful self-assessment questionnaires available to help you determine how healthy your gut is—whether it's functioning full throttle, where the trouble spots are, and whether it's time to worry. I find the Gastrointestinal Health Assessment on the following page from Metagenics particularly useful.

Gastrointestinal Health Assessment

With this questionnaire, you're asked to think back on the last four months and assign a number to a series of questions about gastrointestinal symptoms that you may have experienced (0 = "No or Rarely," 1 = "Occasionally," 4 = "Often," and 8 = "Frequently"). Symptoms are grouped into four categories: gastric function, gastrointestinal inflammation, small intestine and pancreas, and colon. Afterwards, you score yourself to see whether symptoms are low, moderate, or high priority.

GASTROINTESTINAL HEALTH QUESTIONNAIRE

SECTION A

1. Indigestion, food repeats on you after you eat	0	1	4	8
2. Excessive burping, belching and/or bloating following meals	0	1	4	8
3. Stomach spasms and cramping during or after eating	0	1	4	8
4. A sensation that food just sits in your stomach creating uncomfortable fullness, pressure and bloating during or after a meal	0	1	4	8
5. Bad taste in your mouth	0	1	4	8
6. Small amounts of food fill you up immediately	0	1	4	8
7. Skip meals or eat erratically because you have no appetite	0	1	4	8

Total points

SECTION B

1. Strong emotions, or the thought or smell of food aggravates your stomach or makes it hurt	0	1	4	8
2. Feel hungry an hour or two after eating a good-sized meal	0	1	4	8
3. Stomach pain, burning and/or aching over a period of 1–4 hours after eating	0	1	4	8
4. Stomach pain, burning and/or aching relieved by eating food; drinking carbonated beverages, cream or milk; or taking antacids	0	1	4	8
5. Burning sensation in the lower part of your chest, especially when lying down or bending forward	0	1	4	8
6. Digestive problems that subside with rest and relaxation	(No) 0		(Yes) 8	
7. Eating spicy and fatty (fried) foods, chocolate, coffee, alcohol, citrus or hot peppers causes your stomach to burn or ache	0	1	4	8
8. Feel a sense of nausea when you eat	0	1	4	8
9. Difficulty or pain when swallowing food or beverage	0	1	4	8

Total points

SECTION C

1. When massaging under your rib cage on your left side, there is pain, tenderness or soreness   0   1   4   8

2. Indigestion, fullness or tension in your abdomen is delayed, occurring 2-4 hours after eating a meal   0   1   4   8

3. Lower abdominal discomfort is relieved with the passage of gas or with a bowel movement   0   1   4   8

4. Specific foods/beverages aggravate indigestion   0   1   4   8

5. The consistency or form of your stool changes (e.g., from narrow to loose) within the course of a day   0   1   4   8

6. Stool odor is embarrassing   0   1   4   8

7. Undigested food in your stool   0   1   4   8

8. Three or more large bowel movements daily   0   1   4   8

9. Diarrhea (frequent loose, watery stool)   0   1   4   8

10. Bowel movement shortly after eating (within 1 hour)   0   1   4   8

Total points _____

SECTION D

1. Discomfort, pain or cramps in your colon (lower abdominal area)   0   1   4   8

2. Emotional stress and/or eating raw fruits and vegetables causes abdominal bloating, pain, cramps or gas   0   1   4   8

3. Generally constipated (or straining during bowel movements)   0   1   4   8

4. Stool is small, hard and dry   0   1   4   8

5. Pass mucus in your stool   0   1   4   8

6. Alternate between constipation and diarrhea   0   1   4   8

7. Rectal pain, itching or cramping   0   1   4   8

8. No urge to have a bowel movement   (No) 0   (Yes) 8

9. An almost continual need to have a bowel movement   (No) 0   (Yes) 8

Total points _____

Adapted from Gastrointestinal (GI) Health Assessment with permission by Metagenics® 2010.

HEALTH APPRAISAL GRAPH

	LOW PRIORITY			MODERATE PRIORITY				HIGH PRIORITY				Test Score
SECTION A Gastric Function	1	2	3	4	5	6	7	8	20	32	44	56
SECTION B GI Inflammation	1	2	3	4	5	6	7	8	24	40	56	72
SECTION C Small Intestine & Pancreas	2	4	6	8	10	12	14	16	32	48	64	80
SECTION D Colon	2	4	6	8	10	12	14	16	30	44	58	72

Adapted from Gastrointestinal (GI) Health Assessment with permission by Metagenics® 2010.

If you score in the moderate or high range in any category, you may want to discuss the symptoms with your doctor. They may indicate any number of gastrointestinal issues, such as an intolerance or sensitivity to certain foods, acid reflux, or other digestion issues that can often be significantly improved by changing how you eat, when you eat, and what you eat. For more on interpreting your symptoms and how to respond (including red-flag symptoms that should send you to your doctor immediately), consider the following do-it-yourself action guidelines.

DIY Gut Check

As a doctor, I have my own way of determining what may be going on with my patients gut-wise. It's a shorthand method that you can use yourself. Essentially, it requires stepping into my shoes, donning your doctor's cap, and starting to think as I do when a patient comes in to be evaluated for gut issues.

Even if you're feeling fine, doing a regular gut check like this helps you stay on top of potential problems that could be brewing. You may be able to head them off before they become big problems with a simple mealtime makeover or other lifestyle adjustments.

And if you are having symptoms, a gut check can help you decide if you need medical treatment. It also allows you to help your doctor get to the bottom of things faster. The abdomen is a very complicated place, as we've seen, with a lot of organs that perform many functions. Even doctors scratch their heads sometimes trying to figure out what's going on, especially when the only description patients give them is "My stomach hurts." That's why the more specific you can be about the location, severity, type of symptoms, and their duration, the faster you and your doctor can put an end to the problem.

Here are a few questions to ask yourself:

- **Where's the problem located?** Because the abdomen is large and complex, I like to divide this area into quadrants when trying to figure out what's wrong. (See Figure 2 on following page.)

○ *Upper right abdomen.* Pain or sensitivity here can indicate a problem with your liver or gallbladder. If the pain is toward the upper middle part of the abdomen, right underneath the rib cage, it may be related to your stomach or the upper part of your small intestine (called the duodenum). If symptoms are up a bit higher, almost behind the rib cage and sternum (breast bone), you may be suffering from problems in the esophagus.

○ *Upper left abdomen.* Part of your stomach is located in this quadrant, but pain here is rare. When you do have symptoms, they're often related to a spleen problem. This is a good example of an organ that's not part of the digestive system (the spleen belongs to your immune system, helping to fight infections and regulating how much blood is in your body). However, because it sits in the vicinity of your gastrointestinal organs, spleen issues are often mistaken for gut problems.

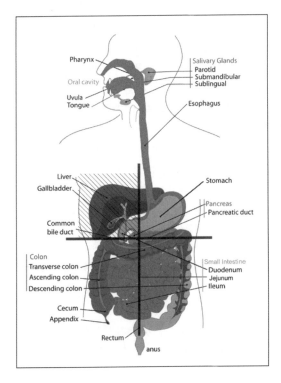

Figure 2.
Abdominal quadrants.
Reprinted from www.clker.com.

○ *Lower right abdomen.* Pain or symptoms in this area are almost invariably related to some issue in the right part of your colon or small intestine. But they can also be signs of a kidney stone or a problem in the right ovary if you're a woman. If pain is toward the middle of the lower abdomen, around the belly button area, it could be a colon problem, as well, or might even be appendicitis, particularly if it comes on suddenly and is severe. And just to complicate things, appendicitis can also be felt elsewhere in many other parts of the abdomen.

○ *Lower left abdomen.* Symptoms here are very common and usually indicate issues with the left part of the colon (though they can also be related to the left kidney or left ovary in women). You see how complicated it gets.

- **What are your symptoms?** Once you know where the pain or discomfort is, think about exactly what you're experiencing. This will allow you to pinpoint even more precisely what could be wrong. For instance, if something's not quite right in the upper middle part of your abdomen and you're experiencing excessive burping or a burning sensation, there's a good chance it's acid reflux. If there's mucus in your stool, and you're alternating between constipation and diarrhea, plus you have lower abdominal cramping, chances are good you may be diagnosed with irritable bowel syndrome. Blood in your stool is also a warning sign. Black blood is generally related to a stomach condition, like an ulcer (certain stomach enzymes turn the blood black). Red blood in the stool is typically a red flag for a colon disorder, such as diverticulitis (pouches in the colon lining that grow weak and bulge out, often causing pain).

- **Have you changed your habits or eating patterns recently?** Not every problem is always what it seems at first. In the above case, for instance, when your stool is red, the culprit may not actually be blood at all, but rather the beets you had for dinner last night. It's a good idea to let your doctor know up front what you've eaten recently and what medications you're taking. It may turn out the irritation in your stomach lining is related to the Advil or aspirin you've been taking for shoulder pain. And if you're skipping meals, chowing down on junk food, and not getting enough fiber from fruits and vegetables, it probably won't surprise your doctor that you're having issues with constipation and bloating, which may or may not be related to a more serious condition.

- **What's your gender?** We all know that men and women are different physically and emotionally. So it shouldn't be a surprise that their digestion is different, too. For example, women secrete less stomach acid than men, and thus suffer from fewer acid-related ulcers. However, their stomachs also empty slower, leading to more nausea and bloating than men. Plus, their colons empty more slowly, causing more constipation. Constipation, related to hormone changes, can intensify during pregnancy and also during menopause. Women also suffer more from gallstones, irritable bowel syndrome, and inflammatory bowel disease. Knowing that your gender can make you more susceptible to issues in certain areas and decrease the likelihood of problems in others also improves the precision of your gut check.

- **How severe and frequent are your symptoms?** We're all exposed to viruses, bacteria, and foods that may create a temporary change in how our digestive system runs. If something is minor, lasts a day, and then it's gone, that's not usually a problem. The time for concern is when you notice a major change that comes on quickly and persists, or one that may be milder but keeps coming back consistently. Any bleeding, severe pain, weight loss, vomiting, or other alarming symptom that doesn't stop is a giant red flag and should send you to your doctor right away. Intermittent or cyclical symptoms usually indicate a chronic condition that's not immediately life-threatening but that may warrant some adjustments in your eating habits, which you and your doctor can discuss.

PARADIGM SHIFT

Too often, modern medicine's approach to gut problems—and most medical maladies, for that matter—is simply to intervene with a pill or a procedure after the damage is done. But that's like pouring thousands of dollars into car repairs that could have been prevented in the first place with some easy, low-cost maintenance. Repairs rarely put your car back into the shape it was, and neither do gut medications and surgery. In fact, they can sometimes make things worse, and often do.

In my experience, the overwhelming majority of people who have gastrointestinal symptoms really just need a lifestyle rearrangement, not surgery or medication. They've stopped taking care of their guts properly, and they need to get back to it again.

And, that's the main message I hope you'll come away with in *No Guts, No Glory*. My Gut Solution plan isn't some pie-in-the-sky-dream diet or ideal lifestyle, but a practical way that you can minimize the damage to your gut that comes from the poor-quality foods, chemical overload, and stress that bombard all of us in the twenty-first century. It's a paradigm shift away from medical treatment toward prevention.

This is a doable plan that can benefit anyone—from those who currently have gut issues and other health problems to those who don't yet and want to keep it that way. If you can contain or prevent the damage by eating better foods most of the time, eliminate the toxins around you and help your liver remove the rest, and maximize your meals by taking digestive enzymes, probiotics, and prebiotics that help you extract more of the nutrients you need, then you're way ahead of the game.

Remember my guarantee from the first chapter—start caring for your gut right now and you'll not only reverse or avoid many illnesses and diseases, but you just might achieve full health and vigor, too. That's the Gut Solution, and that's what we'll begin exploring next. Get ready to learn the specific steps you can take on your journey to optimum wellness.

PART TWO

The Gut Solution

8

The Gut-Smart Eating Plan

Let food be thy medicine, thy medicine shall be thy food.
—HIPPOCRATES (C. 460–377 B.C.)

Let nothing which can be treated by diet
be treated by other means.
—MAIMONIDES (1138–1204 A.D.)

*D*oes this describe you? You get up for work and run out the door without eating breakfast. There just isn't time, and besides you're not that hungry until closer to lunch. One of your coworkers, though, has sprung for donuts, so you grab one at the front desk and finish it off on your way down the hall to your office.

Lunchtime rolls around. Your sugar high from the donut has worn off and you're dragging. But you've got a big deadline, so you run down to the corner deli, grab a soda and chips, then rush back to your desk to work some more. You hardly notice what you're eating. Later in the afternoon, you feel tired again and bloated.

By the time you shut down for the day, it's 6:30. Late again, and no time to cook dinner. You pick up Chinese food on the way home for your family, but no one's home yet from after-school activities and work, so you sit alone eating mindlessly while your thoughts drift back to all that paperwork piled on your desk for tomorrow. Later, as you climb into bed, your stomach is churning and you have the beginnings of a headache. You pop an antacid tablet and vow to begin eating better—and at a more leisurely pace—soon. Maybe when your work load eases up. . . .

The truth is, few of us think much about the way we eat. We swallow our meals down on the run. We give little thought to our food's nutritional content. And we certainly don't pay much attention to whether it sits well in our guts once we've finished everything off. What all this boils down to is one giant problem for our gastrointestinal health and our general well-being.

In this chapter, I hope to convince you why it's so crucial to change your entire approach to selecting, preparing, and eating food—step one of the Gut Solution. What follows are specific guidelines designed to mesh with the intricate biology of your gastrointestinal tract. I call it the Gut-Smart Eating Plan—a two-part strategy that will help improve the way you eat as well as what you eat. Follow it, and I have no doubt you'll notice a dramatic difference in your appreciation of food, your energy levels, and your overall vitality and health.

GUT-SMART EATING STRATEGIES

In medicine there are errors of commission and errors of omission. It sounds complicated, but basically it means that some problems are created by things we do (errors of commission) and some problems are caused by things we fail to do (errors of omission). The gut is a great example of this. We create all kinds of gut snafus when we choose high-density fatty foods and scarf them down without chewing or paying much attention. These are errors of commission—eating habits we hardly think about that wreak widespread gut havoc. We'll discuss errors of omission (such as not eating enough fresh fruits and vegetables and other nutrient-rich foods) later in this chapter. First, though, I want to talk about our growing alienation from food—one of the major errors of commission and the first problem the Gut-Smart Eating Plan is designed to fix.

Improve the Way You Eat by Transforming Your Food M.O.

Most of us don't know much about the foods we feed our bodies. We don't know how they're prepared. We don't cook them properly. And we hardly take time to enjoy them. We've simply lost that loving feeling for our food—to our great detriment.

The good news is this is a fairly easy fix, requiring a few adjustments in your approach to eating. Really, it requires spending a little more time selecting, preparing, appreciating, and savoring your food. What I'm talking about is falling in love with the wonderful ritual of mealtime.

To work right, your gut actually needs a full eating experience, starting with a little predining invitation to begin prepping itself for the arrival of food. It's called the cephalic phase of digestion, which actually starts when you first begin anticipating a meal. The smells and sights of food cooking—even just a momentary craving before you actually begin—prompt your brain and nervous system to signal your stomach and other digestive organs to begin secreting enzymes. Precise signals continue to be sent as you bite, chew, and swallow. For instance, receptors in your mouth work to identify the types of nutrients in your food (like protein or carbohydrates) to ensure that the right enzymes are ready as food moves through the gastrointestinal tract for breakdown.

Once in the stomach, the gastric phase begins. Enzymes continue to be released as needed to digest food, and signals are sent to ready the small intestine for the final leg of the digestive journey—the intestinal phase. The entire process is highly complex, involving organs, enzymes, nerves, hormones, microbes, and blood vessels. Each is necessary, and every phase is intricately connected to the next. Interrupt even one small part, and the effects reverberate throughout your entire gastrointestinal system. For example, key nutrients may fail to be extracted and distributed throughout your body.

It's not too hard to see then that our failure to connect emotionally with our food is hampering our gut's ability to do its job. When you munch packaged nacho chips or gobble down a burger while driving or grab a chocolate bar when you're under stress or eat takeout pizza alone in your den, you deprive your gut of all the necessary preparation it needs to do its digestive work. There are no pre-meal smells, no antic-ipation of delights to come, no savoring of tastes and textures. Only stress, tension, and rushing; only improperly chewed food, missed sig-nals, and indigestion. There's no chance your gut can be fully focused on its digestive duties because there are so many other biologic and physiologic forces overwhelming and disrupting its inner workings.

All this stress and mindless noshing becomes a vicious cycle. Remember how stress triggers ghrelin, the hunger hormone that ups your craving for carbohydrates, sweet treats, and comfort foods? You pack on weight, crave more, and so it goes. And consider this: stud-ies show that a lack of family meals (one result of our busy lifestyles) contributes to childhood obesity (Hammons, 2011). That's because, left to their own devices, kids tend to grab more processed junk foods—something that doesn't happen as often when parents prepare balanced meals and sit down with their kids for some low-stress fam-ily bonding. You can see how our dysfunctional relationship with food—our disregard for how the gut works best—is setting us all up for health troubles in the future.

The bottom line: we've got to change our food M.O. (*modus operandi*). That's a fancy Latin term for mode of operation—mean-ing we've got to change our mealtime habits or manner of eating. We need to reverse our errors of commission and make food a priority. We need to get back to preparing meals from scratch, breathing in the smells, and dining in a tranquil environment that boosts diges-tion rather than undermines it. We've got to start eating in a way that's consistent with the biology of our gut.

Try incorporating these Gut-Smart tips at mealtimes:

• Leave stress, anger, and worry at the dining-room door.

• Make eating special—a ritual. Allow space for meals in your day at consistent times.

- Eat slowly and chew your food thoroughly. Be mindful about what you're eating. Really taste the flavors and enjoy them.

- Eat with family or friends . . . laughing and breaking bread together cuts stress, boosts pleasure, and gets those digestive juices flowing.

- Don't jump right up and rush off afterward. Sit quietly for a while to allow peaceful digestion.

Improve What You Eat with Simple Nutrition Fixes

Remember that saying by Mark Twain, "To eat is human, to digest, divine"? Just because something goes into your mouth doesn't mean your digestive system will break it down properly—or at all. We just saw how our poor approach to dining disrupts the gut's ability to digest what comes in. But if you're not loading your table with foods that contain all the nutrients you need or your gut is unable for any reason to process the nutrients that pass through it, your health will also suffer. In fact, poor food quality is perhaps the main cause of illness in this country today. That's why eating well (or better than you do now) is the second key piece of the Gut-Smart Eating Plan. This may require more thought and effort than changing your food M.O., but altering what you eat so it's more nutritious is well worth it in terms of long-term health benefits.

Just so we're clear: *No Guts, No Glory* isn't a nutrition book. I'm not going to teach you how many calories are in 3 ounces of chicken or how much vitamin C you should get every day. You can consult with your doctor for that or check out one of the many nutrition guides available, including those in the Resources section at the back of this book. But since digesting food is one of your gut's primary roles, it only makes sense that you should think about strategies to help it do its job with optimum efficiency. And as we saw in the last chapter, one way to do that is by feeding your gut the food it was meant to eat: natural, unprocessed foods packed with plenty of nutrients that it evolved over eons to digest. Let me share some simple

Gut-Smart nutrition guidelines that I've found particularly helpful for maximizing gastrointestinal function.

- **Think essential nutrients, not calories.** What matters most to your body isn't the number of calories in your food, but how many and what kinds of nutrients it contains. The more there are and the greater the variety, the better off you'll be.

    There are two major types of nutrients—macronutrients and micronutrients—and you need all of them to be healthy. (See the inset "Essential Nutrients for Life" on page 92.) Each one plays a vital role. Remember those errors of omission (things we fail to do) that hinder or harm our gut's ability to do its work? Omit just a single nutrient (or fall short on requirements or consume low-quality sources), and you can't expect to function at top capacity.

    Macronutrients. There are three types—carbohydrates, proteins, and fats—and you need all of them in your diet to give your body energy.

    ○ Carbohydrates are made up of starches and sugars and are your body's primary fuel source. They're stored in the muscles and liver for use as needed. Look for them mostly in starchy vegetables, grains, fruits, milk, beans and other legumes, and yogurt. Non-starchy vegetables, nuts, and seeds also contain carbohydrates but in smaller quantities.

    ○ Protein is found in meats, poultry, seafood, eggs, cheese, milk, nuts, and beans and other legumes. Certain starchy foods and vegetables also contain some protein. Your body breaks down protein into amino acids and needs a steady supply for tissue repair, immune function, preserving lean muscle mass, making essential hormones and enzymes, and supplying energy when carbohydrates aren't available.

    ○ Fats often get a bad rap for packing on pounds, but you need some for survival. Not only is fat the most concentrated source of energy, but it's also crucial for absorbing certain vitamins, supplying essential fatty acids (including omega-3s and omega-6s), maintaining cell membranes, and assuring normal growth and development. The three main types of dietary fat are saturated fat (found in meat, butter, cream, and other animal-derived products, which should be eaten in limited amounts but not eliminated completely); unsaturated fat (the best kinds are found in nuts, canola oil, olive oil, avocados, and cold-water fish); and trans fat ("bad fats" typically lurking in baked goods, snack foods, and margarine, which should be avoided).

How we're doing: for much of human history, it was a struggle to get the required amounts of proteins, carbohydrates, and fats, but not so today. Given our propensity for comfort foods and haphazard eating, it shouldn't surprise anyone that most of us consume far too many of the wrong kinds of macronutrients and not enough of the right kinds. And we all know the unfortunate results: obesity and poor health. We'll discuss some of the healthiest macronutrient sources in a bit. Be sure to check out the Resources section, too, for more detailed information.

Micronutrients. There are twenty-eight essential vitamins and minerals (plus some likely trace minerals currently being studied, such as vanadium and boron) that your body needs to function but can't manufacture itself. It gets them from macronutrient food sources. They're called *micro*nutrients because you require smaller amounts than the macronutrients. However, they're every bit as important. In fact, you couldn't metabolize macronutrients without them.

How we're doing: the dearth of high-quality macronutrients in our diet is also starving us of essential micronutrients. In fact, up to 75 percent of us aren't getting enough vitamins and minerals like iron, vitamins B_6 and B_{12}, folic acid, and zinc. It's not that we have full-blown vitamin deficiencies such as pellagra (caused by a lack of niacin), scurvy (caused by a lack of vitamin C), or rickets (caused by a lack of vitamin D). Most of us are getting the minimum required amounts to prevent deficiency diseases. But we're not getting the optimum amount that will bring each of us to full health. We're simply not consuming enough micronutrients to be truly well, and may be setting ourselves up for disease down the road.

One recent study of adolescents who ate a Western diet low in fruits, vegetables, and whole grains (meaning few omega-3 fatty acids and essential micronutrients like folate, a naturally occurring form of folic acid) illustrates the relationship between low vitamin intake and poor health (Howard, 2011). They were likelier to be diagnosed with ADHD than kids with more nutrient-rich diets.

The bottom line: you have the best chance of getting a balance of essential micronutrients by eating the freshest, most nutritious foods possible whenever you can.

ESSENTIAL NUTRIENTS FOR LIFE

Macronutrients

Carbohydrates

Proteins (including essential amino acids)

Fats (including essential fatty acids)

Micronutrients

VITAMINS

Vitamin A

Vitamin B-complex

Thiamine (B_1)

Riboflavin (B_2)

Niacin (B_3)

Pantothenic acid (B_5)

Pyridoxine (B_6)

Folic acid (B_9)

Cyanocobalamin (B_{12})

Biotin

Choline

Vitamin C

Vitamin D

Vitamin E

Vitamin K

MINERALS

Calcium

Chloride

Chromium

Copper

Iodine

Iron

Magnesium

Manganese

Molybdenum

Phosphorus

Potassium

Selenium

Sodium

Zinc

- **Tailor nutrients to your needs.** Again, I'm not going to tell you whether to consume 5,000 international units (IUs) or 10,000 IUs of vitamin D a day or how much protein to eat at dinner. The amount you need depends on your age, gender, stress level, the amount of exercise you do, or whether you're recovering from an illness or surgery. It's very person specific.

  Plus, the recommended amounts will surely keep evolving as more studies come along—and they *will* keep coming because discovering optimum nutrient levels for health is the main challenge in nutrition today.

  The list of nutrients needed may expand, too. For instance, newer research suggests there may be a few "age-essential" micronutrients that older bodies need in greater amounts. Two leading candidates are L-carnitine (made naturally from amino acids in the body) and alpha lipoic acid (a fatty acid found naturally in all cells).

  My advice is, don't change the amounts or types of nutrients you consume based on each new study. I certainly don't. But don't get stuck on one amount or one type either. Just because someone told you ten years ago that rice crackers are the best source of carbohydrates or that 2,000 milligrams (mg) a day of vitamin C is ideal, doesn't mean you should stick with that plan forever. New recommendations do come along every few years, backed by lots of science, so you'll want to stay flexible and open to new findings.

- **Think nonessential nutrients, too.** Yet another reason to eat plenty of fresh fruits and vegetables, beans and other legumes, whole grains, and other plant foods is because they also contain potent disease fighters called phytonutrients. These nutrients work in various ways, including as antioxidants, which protect you against disease-causing cell damage by free radicals that form when you're exposed to environmental contaminants, as well as during the course of your body's normal metabolism. We'll discuss antioxidants and free radicals more in the next chapter.

Just one small example is broccoli. Researchers have found that it and other cruciferous vegetables (those in the cabbage family, including cauliflower and brussels sprouts) are rich in sulforaphane. This unique phytochemical has antioxidant properties that appear to target and kill cancer cells while leaving normal healthy cells alone.

To get the most benefit you can from this substance, though, you'll want your gut—specifically your intestinal bacteria—to be in tip-top shape. They're the ones that actually break down glucoraphanin, which helps form sulforaphane and aid in its distribution throughout the body. Interestingly, sulforaphane even helps keep your gut in good condition. Its antibacterial properties protect against infection with the *H. pylori* bacteria responsible for stomach ulcers and cancer.

- **Eat raw or lightly cooked foods.** The human gut evolved to eat mostly fresh, uncooked foods—living foods. They're readily digestible, and even digest themselves. Think of an apple left on the counter. Within days, it turns brown and shrivels up (self digestion). That's because it contains active enzymes. Foods that are heavily cooked or processed lose these enzymes and are therefore harder for your gut to break down—meaning you don't get all the nutrients available. Raw and lightly cooked foods (those steamed or cooked at low temperatures, rather than fried in oil or flame-broiled, etc.) retain active enzymes and work with your gut's enzymes to thoroughly break down food and extract more nutrients. Almost all raw plant foods, meats, and dairy products contain enzymes. Particularly rich sources include pineapple, papaya, mangos, grapes, avocados, raw honey, unrefined oils, and sprouts.

- **Think pesticide-free, local, and seasonal.** Again, the closer you can get to the way humans used to eat, the better your gut will work. And what could be closer to our ancestors' diet than to eat locally grown, seasonal, and organic foods (grown without the use of synthetic pesticides, fertilizers, or other chemicals)? Look for these Gut-Smart choices at your grocery store or farmers' market. Better yet, head out to a local organic farm, join a CSA (community supported agriculture), or grow your own.

- **Avoid high-glycemic carbs.** These are refined carbohydrates—like white bread, pasta, pastries, and chips—that are rapidly digested by your gut and absorbed, causing a spike in blood sugar and insulin. This can lead to insulin resistance, diabetes, and heart disease. Most of these foods also contain little fiber, few nutrients, and more calories—another error of omission and obstacle to gut health. Opt instead for low-glycemic choices, such as many fresh fruits and vegetables, and whole grains (see the Resources for sources of good choices).

- **Be on alert for food allergies and intolerances.** Some of you may already know you have reactions to certain foods such as those we discussed in Chapter 5. If you suffer from a food allergy, for example, no doubt you've already consulted your doctor. You do your best to avoid the offending foods that put your immune system in attack mode and take care to look out for hidden ingredients that trigger reactions.

  For those with food intolerances, though, things may not be quite so easy or clear. Intolerances are usually caused by a genetic lack of certain enzymes needed to digest specific foods, like gluten, and don't typically produce life-threatening reactions. Rather, intolerances sneak up on you well after you eat a trigger food. Symptoms may include bloating, gaseousness, constipation, and other problems.

  The fact is, a majority of us are lactose intolerant and an increasing number are gluten sensitive, though we may not realize it. Also on the rise are sensitivities to coffee and fructose (particularly when consumed in high amounts, such as in foods and beverages containing high-fructose corn syrup). Remember the Gastro-intestinal Health Assessment questionnaire from the previous chapter? If you scored in the moderate-to-high range for gut symptoms, you may have an intolerance or sensitivity to certain foods. Start paying attention and be aware of how you feel, not minutes after eating, but hours later.

- **Eliminate foods that cause gut issues and choose better types.** If you already know you have food allergies or intolerances, you'll definitely want to start eliminating foods that aggravate symptoms and opt for problem-free, healthier alternatives. And even if you are not experiencing noticeable symptoms or only occasional minor ones, you might also want to begin avoiding potentially trouble-some foods, at least for a while, to test whether you detect a dif-ference or feel better without them. The results may just surprise you. Recent findings show that patients with celiac disease (gluten intolerance) who did not report symptoms and continued eating gluten, nevertheless were found to have under-the-radar symptoms that subsided when they switched to a gluten-free diet and improved their general health (Kurppa, 2011).

  How you choose to eliminate problem foods is up to you, but you'll probably want to do it in conjunction with your doctor. Examples of how to carry out an elimination diet can be found in the Resources section. Some of you might want to try detoxifica-tion and fasting, then eliminating everything at once. Others may find it hard to stop their eating habits cold turkey and will opt for a more gradual elimination. That part is up to you. We'll talk more about detoxification and fasting in the next chapter.

  What follows is by no means a comprehensive list, but it will give you a general idea of trigger foods that can block your gut from full digestion as well as better options that promote gut health. If you have food allergies or intolerances, you'll want to follow these guidelines rigorously. (An asterisk indicates the most common sources of food allergies.) If you don't, eliminating or even just reducing potential culprits in the following categories will likely boost your health and well-being:

◦ *Dairy products.* Avoid: cow's milk*, cream, cream cheese, processed cheeses, and those made with cow's milk. Switch to: almond milk, coconut milk, goat milk, hemp milk, rice milk, and soy milk, non-processed cheeses made without cow's milk, and kefir (a milk drink—also choose brands made without cow's milk).

◦ *Protein.* Avoid: hormone- and antibiotic-fed meats and poultry, processed cold cuts, canned meats, farm-raised seafood (especially shellfish*). Switch to: free-range meats and poultry, wild game, wild-caught seafood, and vegetarian protein sources, including tofu and other soy-based meat substitutes (some people may be soy* sensitive), nuts (some people may be allergic, especially to peanuts*), seeds, and beans and other legumes.

◦ *Grains.* Avoid: high-gluten grains, such as wheat*, barley, oats, and rye. Switch to: buckwheat, millet, quinoa, amaranth, and rice (all are good low-glycemic carbs, by the way).

◦ *Sugars and sweeteners.* Avoid: foods and beverages with added sugar or high-fructose corn syrup, dried fruits, and preserves and jellies. Switch to: fresh fruits, berries, dates, and prunes, raw honey, stevia, and maple syrup.

• **Remember, variety is the spice of life.** We all get in food ruts. We have particular treats we like—favorite foods for breakfast, lunch, and dinner—and we tend to stick with them. Unfortunately, that's not usually a prescription for getting all the macronutrients and micronutrients you need (yes, another error of omission). You have to vary and expand your diet to make sure you're consuming the balance your body requires. You may feel well, but you can't be truly well if you only eat asparagus and broccoli and no other vegetables, or if you stick with apples and oranges to the exclusion of any other fruits.

You have to educate yourself about the many choices available.

Leave your comfort zone. Try bok choy and brussels sprouts. Sample the huckleberries and kiwis. Experiment with flaxseeds or ocean-fresh mahi-mahi. There's a world of tasty and nutritious choices out there. Your gut will work better if it gets nutrients from a wide assortment of wholesome foods, and so will you.

A MATTER OF CHOICE

I know what you're thinking: this all sounds like a lot of work. Okay, I'm not going to lie. My suggestions about changing your approach to food may run contrary to how you eat now. And for some, it may be a really radical departure. Expect a little discomfort in the beginning as you try out the Gut-Smart Eating Plan.

Believe me, I understand. Old habits die hard. I know it's easier to throw a prepared meal into the microwave than to cook up a homemade meal from scratch. A lot of processed foods really are more convenient, they're tastier (given the fact that we're used to them), and they're often less expensive. Let's face it, salmon and broccoli cost a lot more than a Happy Meal.

But just because it's hard to make time for meals and to properly nourish yourself doesn't mean you shouldn't try. Actually, there are many fresh, nutritious foods that are quite budget-friendly, and finding them is more doable than you think. But as we've seen in this chapter, you may have to stretch yourself a little in the beginning as you learn about healthier choices and seek them out. Sure, you can let yourself off the hook and continue starving your body with on-the-run noshing and low-nutrient choices. No one has a pistol to your head. You're free to live and eat as you choose. But as I tell my patients, there will be a price to pay for choosing to ignore your gut health. It's as simple as that. Fill yourself up day after day with soda, hoagies, and nacho chips, and your health will never be what it could be.

The bottom line: choose wisely. You can't be truly well without giving your gut adequate preparation to get the digestion wheels turning and feeding it nutrient-rich foods—and worst-case scenario, your health will decline. Just ask the tens of millions of Americans who buy antacids or take the "purple pill" (Nexium) for acid reflux. What they didn't realize is they had a choice. As an old Chinese proverb notes, "He that takes medicine and neglects diet, wastes the skill of the physician." That's along the lines of our common saying: "An ounce of prevention is worth a pound of cure." It's so much easier, cheaper, and way more pleasant to enhance your gut's performance and function rather than invest in treatments for gut issues.

If your gut seems to be functioning well right now, congratulations, you still have a choice. But just because you feel well today, doesn't mean you really are. Remember that few of us eat like we should day in and day out, year after year for a lifetime. At some point, those rushed meals of processed, chemical-laden foods (even if you keep them to a minimum) are likely to catch up with you. And don't forget the world itself is laden with toxic chemicals that further mess with your gut's capacity to function. You may still have time, but once illness or dysfunction sets in, your choices get taken away. Making some changes now to your food M.O. and selecting more nutritious foods is similar to taking out an insurance policy that will pay major dividends down the line. You may just end up with the best health you've ever had!

And if you do have some gut issues, don't worry. Making some changes now can often reverse these problems without the need for costly medications that may cause additional problems. If you don't want your gut to continue being the limiting factor that blocks you from wellness, a Gut-Smart makeover is definitely in order.

Yes, it will require some effort, especially at first. But it will get easier. I promise. In fact, I'm certain the immediate boost in your digestion and health will be all the motivation you need to keep going until mindful eating and good food choices become second nature.

Next, we'll explore another key piece of the Gut Solution—how to further enhance your wellness by boosting your gut's ability to detoxify your body of harmful substances and get rid of waste.

9

Detoxification

What fools indeed we mortals are
To lavish care upon a car
With ne'er a bit of time to see
About our own machinery!

—JOHN KENDRICK BANGS (1862–1922)

*M*ost of us walk through our days blissfully ignorant about all the potentially hazardous things that make their way into our bodies. There's that juicy green apple you enjoyed for a snack in the afternoon. Chances are it harbors pesticide residues. That glass of tap water you drank after lunch may contain dozens of chemicals, including arsenic. The air you breathe every day could be polluted with ozone and other hazardous toxins, particularly if you're an urban dweller. Even your shampoo and glass cleaner probably carry a list of chemicals on the label that you can't even pronounce and certainly don't want inside you.

The more hazardous substances we encounter, the harder our bodies have to work and the harder it is to get rid of everything. We get overloaded, as we saw in Chapter 6. The proof may be in the amount of cancer we see, chronic fatigue, degenerative disorders like arthritis, and maybe even Alzheimer's and other brain conditions. It's hard to prove that toxins actually cause illness. But you can be sure they're not helping your body function. Just as your car engine needs clean gasoline to run optimally, your body also needs a clean operating system for full health. All these substances are obviously dirtying up your internal machinery—and likely robbing you of your vitality and vibrancy.

Nor are chemicals the only assaults that come our way every day. Think about the constant stress we're under and the medicines we take for various ailments and discomforts, as well as the alcohol, cigarettes, and drugs we may use to calm down or help us sleep. Granted, we have more control over our exposure to these, but it can still be hard for some of us to avoid them entirely.

My point is that good gut health doesn't just come from eliminating toxic foods and those that trigger allergies and intolerances or by enjoying a deeper relationship with our food (all of which we explored in the last chapter). Promoting a healthy gut is also about giving your gastrointestinal system as much of a break as possible from the continual barrage of modern dangers and psychological toxins and assisting it in eliminating the inevitable harmful substances that do find their way in.

This is the second step of the Gut Solution—Detoxification—and at the heart of this process is the liver, the remarkable gut organ that oversees clearing out dangerous chemicals and other hazardous elements from your body. I'm going to show you how to assist it in its critical detoxification duties by making lifestyle changes and feeding it and the rest of your detox system a steady supply of crucial nutrients.

GUT INTEGRITY

Recall how your gut evolved to eat natural foods that were plentiful in the wild throughout much of human history. Well, it also evolved to handle toxins when the world was still relatively free of chemicals, pollutants, greenhouse gases, and unrelenting stress. Unfortunately, that world doesn't exist anymore, and your detoxification system simply hasn't caught up yet—if it ever actually could.

Many of these toxins are man-made. They don't exist naturally in nature, and our bodies were never meant to handle them. Nor were we designed to move at the high-speed pace of twenty-first century life. Remember that list of things that can block our ability to detoxify and degrade our overall health:

- Chemicals, heavy metals, and other pollutants from household and personal care products, and in our food, air, and drinking water

- Chronic stress

- Alcohol, tobacco, and drugs

- Prescription and over-the-counter medications

- Sleep deprivation

- Lack of exercise

- Normal metabolic wastes created after cells take in oxygen and nutrients

The harm being done to your gut and other organs can't be seen with the naked eye. Rather, you would need to peer at their fundamental structure through an electron microscope. That's where the damage occurs—on the cellular level—quietly assaulting their integrity. Incidentally, your body's other detoxification pathways (respiratory system, urinary tract, and skin) also face similar troubles. Ultimately, every part of you suffers.

The real problem centers on what are known as free radicals. These are unstable atoms and molecules that are created by environmental contaminants, stress, cigarette smoke, and even oxygen metabolism inside you. Once unleashed, they cause oxidative damage to your body's cells. In fact, they're believed to be behind most chronic diseases (including cancer and many other preventable conditions) and may accelerate the aging process.

Normally, your body deals with these tiny health terrorists by releasing a supply of free-radical fighters called antioxidants (including essential vitamins like C and E as well as other nutrients). But when the body is overrun with more toxins than it can process or you don't eat enough antioxidant-rich foods to ward off the extra load of free radicals, damage occurs. Your gut—and liver in particular—may be especially hard hit by free-radical injury because they're in direct contact with so many harmful substances.

DETOX CENTRAL

How do you protect your body from free radicals and more effectively eliminate all the things that cause them to form? So much boils down to the health of your liver. As your body's largest organ, the liver is one of the busiest workhorses around. In its detoxification role, it separates out the good substances that enter your body from the bad, and sees that the dangerous things are neutralized and eliminated before they have a chance to hurt your health.

It does this in two phases. In phase one, harmful fat-soluble toxins that filter through your liver in your blood are transformed into intermediate compounds through a complex biochemical process that involves several enzymes. Sometimes these new compounds are more toxic than their original forms, even carcinogenic. But this necessary in-between step makes it easier to finish transforming them into non-dangerous compounds in the second phase. Interestingly, one of the byproducts of this transformation is—you guessed it—free radicals.

When everything is working right, these free radicals are easily handled as antioxidants rush in to reduce their capacity for damage. Your liver can then move to phase two where it secretes more enzymes (in a process called conjugation) that bind the dangerous intermediate compounds to nontoxic water-soluble molecules. These harmless substances are then easily excreted by your kidneys as urine or mixed with bile and eliminated in your feces.

You can see why it's absolutely crucial that your cleanser-in-chief be in top shape. If your liver enzymes are disrupted during either of these two phases—by, say, an overload of toxins or liver injury—dangerous compounds might not be rendered harmless. Instead, they're likely to end up staying in your body doing serious damage to everything in their path.

One example is when harmful gut bacteria produce an enzyme called beta-glucuronidase, which blocks an important substance called glucuronic acid. Glucuronic acid is needed during phase two to neutralize certain toxins and hormones so they can be eliminated through your urine and feces. Without it, these toxins are reabsorbed and increase your risk of colon cancer and possibly other cancers. All in all, when your liver can't perform its two-step detox operation, it's a prescription for health disaster in nearly every system of your body.

One way to assess how well your liver is cleansing your body is to have your doctor test its detoxification capabilities. There are a few different types of liver function challenge tests (also called functional liver detoxification profiles). These differ from a regular liver function test (mentioned in Chapter 5), which involves conducting a group of blood tests to look for evidence of liver disease. In contrast, a challenge test may require ingesting substances that the liver usually processes (like acetaminophen, for instance) and then examining your urine and saliva to see if it was excreted properly.

Another way to assess whether your liver may be falling short in its detox duties is by filling out a self-assessment questionnaire that can help you pinpoint signs of a high toxic load in your body. One that I find especially useful is the Detoxification Questionnaire from Metagenics (see following page).

Detoxification Questionnaire

With this questionnaire, you're asked to assign a number value to symptoms you may be having in each major organ system, as well as rate your emotional well-being, energy levels, and other health indicators (0 = "Never or almost never have symptom," 1 = "Occasionally have symptom but effect isn't severe," 2 = "Occasionally have symptom and effect is severe," 3 = "Frequently have symptom but effect isn't severe," and 4 = "Frequently have symptom and effect is severe").

MEDICAL SYMPTOMS QUESTIONNAIRE

HEAD

Headaches _____

Faintness _____

Dizziness _____

Insomnia _____

Total _____

EYES

Watery or itchy eyes _____

Swollen, reddened or sticky
eyelids _____

Bags or dark circles under eyes _____

Blurred or tunnel vision _____

Total _____

EARS

Itchy ears _____

Earaches, ear infections _____

Drainage from ear _____

Ringing in ears, hearing loss _____

Total _____

NOSE

Stuffy nose _____

Sinus problems _____

Hay fever _____

Sneezing attacks _____

Excessive mucus formation _____

Total _____

MOUTH/THROAT

Chronic coughing _____

Gagging, frequent need to clear throat _____

Sore throat, hoarseness, loss of voice _____

Swollen or discolored tongue,
gums, lips _____

Canker sores _____

Total _____

SKIN

Acne _____

Hives, rashes, dry skin _____

Hair loss _____

Flushing, hot flashes _____

Excessive sweating _____

Total _____

HEART

Chest pain _____

Irregular or skipped heartbeat _____

Rapid or pounding heartbeat _____

Total _____

LUNGS

Chest congestion _____

Asthma, bronchitis _____

Shortness of breath _____

Difficulty breathing _____

Total _____

DIGESTIVE TRACT

Nausea, vomiting _____

Diarrhea _____

Constipation _____

Bloated feeling _____

Belching, passing gas _____

Heartburn _____

Intestinal/stomach pain _____

Total _____

JOINTS/MUSCLE

Pain or aches in joints _____

Arthritis _____

Stiffness or limitation of movement _____

Feeling of weakness or tiredness _____

Pain or aches in muscles _____

Total _____

WEIGHT

Binge eating/drinking _____

Craving certain foods _____

Excessive weight _____

Water retention _____

Underweight _____

Compulsive eating _____

Total _____

ENERGY/ACTIVITY

Fatigue, sluggishness _____

Apathy, lethargy _____

Hyperactivity _____

Restlessness _____

Total _____

MIND

Poor memory _____

Confusion, poor comprehension _____

Difficulty in making decisions _____

Stuttering or stammering _____

Slurred speech _____

Learning disabilities _____

Poor concentration _____

Poor physical coordination _____

Total _____

EMOTIONS

Mood swings _____

Anxiety, fear, nervousness _____

Anger, irritability, aggressiveness _____

Depression _____

Total _____

OTHER

Frequent illness _____

Frequent or urgent urination _____

Genital itch or discharge _____

Total _____

GRAND TOTAL _____

Adapted from Detoxification Questionnaire
with permission by Metagenics®2005.

Next you answer a series of questions about the kinds of substances you typically ingest, including prescription and over-the-counter drugs, alcohol, and tobacco, as well as your personal history with allergies, chemical sensitivities, and other conditions. These answers are also assigned a value.

XENOBIOTIC TOLERABILITY

1. Are you presently using prescription drugs?
   ❏ Yes (1 pt.)   ❏ No (0 pt.)
   If yes, how many are you currently taking?
   _____ (1 pt. each)

2. Are you presently taking one or more of the following over-the-counter drugs?
   ❏ Cimetidine (2 pts.)
   ❏ Acetaminophen (2 pts.)
   ❏ Estradiol (2 pts.)

3. If you have used or currently use prescription drugs, which of the following scenarios best represents your response to them:
   ❏ Experience side effects, drug(s) is (are) efficacious at lowered dose(s) (3 pts.)
   ❏ Experience side effects, drug(s) is (are) efficacious at usual dose(s) (2 pts.)
   ❏ Experience no side effects, drug(s) is (are) usually not efficacious (2 pts.)
   ❏ Experience no side effects, drug(s) is (are) usually efficacious (0 pt.)

4. Do you currently use or within the last 6 months had you regularly used tobacco products?
   ❏ Yes (2 pts.)   ❏ No (0 pt.)

5. Do you have strong negative reactions to caffeine or caffeine containing products?
   ❏ Yes (1 pt.)   ❏ No (0 pt.)
   ❏ Don't know (0 pt.)

6. Do you commonly experience "brain fog," fatigue, or drowsiness?
   ❏ Yes (1 pt.)   ❏ No (0 pt.)

7. Do you develop symptoms on exposure to fragrances, exhaust fumes, or strong odors?
   ❏ Yes (1 pt.)   ❏ No (0 pt.)
   ❏ Don't know (0 pt.)

8. Do you feel ill after you consume even small amounts of alcohol?
   ❏ Yes (1 pt.)   ❏ No (0 pt.)
   ❏ Don't know (0 pt.)

9. Do you have a personal history of
   ❏ Environmental and/or chemical sensitivities (5 pts.)
   ❏ Chronic fatigue syndrome (5 pts.)
   ❏ Multiple chemical sensitivity (5 pts.)
   ❏ Fibromyalgia (3 pts.)
   ❏ Parkinson's type symptoms (3 pts.)
   ❏ Alcohol or chemical dependence (2 pts.)
   ❏ Asthma (1 pt.)

10. Do you have a history of significant exposure to harmful chemicals such as herbicides, insecticides, pesticides, or organic solvents?
    ❏ Yes (1 pt.)   ❏ No (0 pt.)

11. Do you have an adverse or allergic reaction when you consume sulfite-containing foods such as wine, dried fruit, salad bar vegetables, etc?
    ❏ Yes (1 pt.)   ❏ No (0 pt.)
    ❏ Don't know (0 pt.)

GRAND TOTAL: _____

Adapted from Detoxification Questionnaire with permission by Metagenics®2005.

A high total score (greater than 50 for the symptom questions and greater than 10 for the questions about substances you ingest and typical reactions) indicates you may have a large toxic load—meaning your liver could be injured or overwhelmed. A moderate score (15–49 on the symptom portion and 5–9 for the substances/reactions questions) also indicates your liver may not be functioning as well as it could.

DETOX STRATEGIES

So what do you do if you score high or in the moderate range? Obviously, it's time to begin assisting your liver, by boosting its ability to morph dangerous chemicals into benign throwaways. And that's what this second step of the Gut Solution is really about—helping your detox organs eliminate problem substances with optimum efficiency so you can enjoy full health and optimum well-being.

There are many excellent detoxification programs out there. Most put participants through an intense regimen that lasts for a set period of time (for example, ten days or twenty-eight days). During this time, you start with a clearing phase where you eliminate potential allergenic foods and add nutritional supports and other lifestyle changes that encourage detoxification. Then you reintroduce some of the foods as you prepare to step back into real life. A few approaches also involve various levels of fasting, modified fasting, or juicing, as well as colon cleanses (similar to an enema but with herbal liquids instead of water).

In general, I don't think it's necessary for everyone to go through one of these formal detox programs. Don't get me wrong; they're not likely to be harmful (although, in the case of colon cleanses, there's very little science to support their use). I've known plenty of people who feel dramatically energized after participating in one, and I'm all for that. Some of us need a more radical start to mark the beginning of our new lifestyle. We want a clear break from our old habits, and that's perfectly okay . . . as long as we don't delude ourselves that we can go back to our old way of life and maintain all the positive health improvements we've initiated.

But the fact is, detoxification doesn't just happen during a single week every ten years. It's got to become a lifelong habit, part of your daily health regimen. And that's the thrust of my message in *No Guts, No Glory*. Essentially, my detoxification plan involves many of the same steps as more formal detox programs, except that you can begin following my recommendations right now, adding them into your life in a way that works for you.

You start by eliminating foods that harm your gut—those containing refined sugars, artificial colorings, pesticides, and other problem substances. We discussed some of these strategies in the last chapter, and we'll look at some more in this one. We'll also explore ways to reduce environmental toxins as much as possible and add supplements and functional foods to your diet that protect your liver from free-radical damage and enhance its ability to do the detoxing for you. Check the Resources in the back of the book, too, for more information about making detoxification a part of your life.

Eliminate What Ails Your Gut

- **Reduce everyday harm.** Read labels when you shop for cleaning products, shampoo, toothpaste, food, house paint, furniture, plastic cookware, and pretty much anything else you use in your everyday life. Most contain hazardous chemicals that drive up your toxic body burden. Consider buying "green" alternatives that harbor few or no toxins. This includes selecting organically grown fresh vegetables and fruits whenever you can to cut your consumption of pesticides and herbicides. If you can't go organic, be sure to wash produce thoroughly. Also, buy meats, chicken, and seafood from animals that aren't fed hormones or antibiotics. You won't be able to rid your life of every hazardous substance, but you can cut the amount that your liver has to contend with. Every little bit helps.

- **Lay off alcohol, tobacco, and drugs.** Tobacco and recreational drugs are absolute no-no's when it comes to gut health—both can lead to serious gastrointestinal disorders (not to mention disorders throughout your entire body). So can alcohol, a particular problem for your liver if you overindulge. However, an occasional drink can be fun and relaxing, and probably won't hurt your gut if done in moderation. If you're addicted to any of these substances, be sure you seek help. See the Resources for more on breaking addictions.

- **Take a stress break.** I know this is easier said than done, but it's critical to protect your gut from the chaos of modern life. Ongoing stress signals from the brain are behind all sorts of gastrointestinal upsets. Stress boosts your cravings for junk food that hinders proper gut function and packs on the pounds, plus it increases the likelihood that you may turn to addictive substances, like alcohol and cigarettes. In turn, the rising toxic load as you attempt to deal with stress adds even more stress to your body. Figure out what's causing the stress, avoid situations and people that add to your anxiety level, and look for healthier ways to cope. Exercise, meditation, getting together with friends, listening to music, watching a movie, taking a warm bath, and journaling are all good outlets when life spirals out of control. Find what works for you and try scheduling some down time every day. Also consider giving up stimulants like caffeine.

- **Cut down on medications.** Maybe you need to take pharmaceutical drugs for a particular illness, and can't cut down or stop taking them. That's okay. Your liver is the chief processor of drugs and should be able to handle a reasonable amount, especially if you boost its health. You might also talk with your doctor about alternative medications that are easier on your gut.

  What you do have control over, though, is how many over-the-counter drugs you take. Consider easing up on gut-injuring medications like NSAID painkillers, which can irritate the stomach lining and lead to ulcers, as well as antacids, which often lead to constipation and promote overgrowth of bad gut bacteria. The fewer substances you thrust on your gut, the better it will operate.

Adopt Gut-Promoting Detox Habits

- **Eat more fiber.** This means more plant foods, including green vegetables, bran, beans and peas, brown rice, and nuts and seeds. Interestingly, most of the fiber you eat is roughage (stems and skin) that isn't digested. But it's incredibly important for detoxification because it adds bulk to your stool and holds moisture to help move waste through your colon and out of your body. As an added bonus, it makes you feel full so you don't eat as much or the wrong kinds of food!

- **Drink water . . . then drink some more.** Keep yourself hydrated with tap, distilled, filtered, or non-carbonated mineral water—at least two quarts a day—to help ferry nutrients into cells and aid your liver, colon, and kidneys as they flush toxins from your body. Drinking a cup of warm lemon water daily can relieve gut problems like constipation, heartburn, and nausea. What's more, it promotes bile production in the liver and cleanses the gallbladder, further helping digestion and elimination of wastes. Plus, the acid in lemons also keeps down the growth of unhealthy gut bacteria.

- **Exercise regularly.** Working out brings more oxygen to your body's tissues and organs (including gut organs) so they function more effectively. It also burns fat, which reduces the amount of storage area available for fat-soluble toxins. Studies show that when you get moving, so does waste in your colon, preventing constipation and aiding in swifter excretion of toxins. Pick physical activities you like to do, whether it's yoga, riding a bike, or just walking, and do them regularly.

- **Sleep more—and better.** Lack of sleep causes a disruption of hunger hormones that signal your brain that you need to eat more. Unfortunately, the foods you end up craving are usually chemical-laden junk foods that unleash more toxins into your body.

    Nipping stress in the bud and working out should help promote better sleep. But you can also try other sleep inducements such as reading quietly instead of watching TV before turning out the lights; keeping your room dark and cool; avoiding stimulants like caffeine and nicotine; and trying natural sleep remedies when insomnia gets the better of you, like magnesium supplements or a hot lavender oil bath before bedtime.

Take Detox-Promoting Nutrients

One way to keep your liver's integrity intact is by feeding it nutrients that protect it from toxins and free-radical damage as well as boost its ability to function at the top of its game. Because your body does not manufacture all the nutrients and antioxidants (free-radical scavengers) it needs, you'll want to provide a steady supply in your diet. All the more reason to follow the Gut-Smart Eating Plan with its emphasis on fresh, nutrient-rich functional foods. However, even if your meals include a lot of these foods, chances are you're not consistently getting enough of them to make a real difference. For this reason, you may want to also take daily supplements as part of your detoxification lifestyle. Here's my list of recommended detox-promoting vitamins, minerals, amino acids, and special plant nutrients:

- **L-glutathione.** Some people call this the master antioxidant because it's contained in every cell of your body and is crucial to fighting off free-radical damage from contaminants and a toxic lifestyle. Your liver contains the highest levels of L-glutathione in your body to help it contend with the high load of harmful substances it meets on a daily basis. Not only does this amino acid destroy free radicals in phase one of detoxification, but it also helps convert toxins, like heavy metals and pesticides, to less dangerous water-soluble chemicals during phase two. Plus, it gives a boost to other antioxidants so they work more efficiently.

  If you're low in L-glutathione (and many people are, especially as they age) or your liver is overwhelmed by toxins and your L-glutathione stores can't keep pace (also a problem for millions of

Americans), your body simply won't be cleansed properly. All *raw* fruits and vegetables contain L-glutathione, but particularly good sources include asparagus, avocados, broccoli, and spinach, as well as garlic and fresh meats, poultry, and fish. So be sure to add more of these at meal times in addition to taking supplements. One supplement that I really like is GlutaClear from Metagenics, which helps boost the body's store of L-glutathione.

- **Essential vitamins and minerals.** Remember that list of essential micronutrients from the last chapter? Well, many of those are also essential antioxidants, including vitamins A, C, E, and selenium. Not only do they work to fight free radicals, but they also help your body produce and synthesize L-glutathione to promote greater liver function. Adequate stores of B vitamins, including vitamins B_1, B_6, folic acid, B_{12}, and riboflavin, are also important in keeping L-glutathione levels where they need to be. Since your body needs a constant influx of these nutrients, eating plenty of fresh vegetables and fruits, nuts and seeds, grains, beans and other legumes, and some meats, poultry, and fish, as well as taking a comprehensive multivitamin, should give you the necessary balance to keep your free-radical defenses working well.

- **L-glutamine.** This amino acid antioxidant helps your liver manufacture and store L-glutathione. In addition to taking a supplement, you may want to include more L-glutamine-rich foods in your diet, including beef, fish, beans and other legumes, chicken, and dairy products.

- **L-cysteine.** This is yet another important amino acid and antioxidant that also aids your liver in producing L-glutathione and detoxifying your body. It's also found in high-protein foods, like poultry, eggs, wheat, and dairy products, and is available in supplement form. However, because L-cysteine is not easily absorbed by your body, you may want to take N-acetylcysteine (NAC) instead. This altered form of L-cysteine isn't found in foods, but the supplements are water soluble and are believed to be more readily usable in the body. NAC is particularly effective at protecting your liver against the effects of acetaminophen, alcohol, and environmental pollutants.

- **L-taurine.** Also derived from L-cysteine, this amino acid is a key ingredient in bile acids that help break down fats and remove toxins via your feces. Some evidence suggests that supplementing with L-taurine may also prevent fat buildup in the liver. In addition, it's a potent antioxidant that aids your liver's detoxification ability. Like L-cysteine, it's available in protein-rich foods.

- **Flavonoids.** These chemical compounds found naturally in plants aren't considered essential nutrients, but they should be as far as I'm concerned. Flavonoids—also called phytonutrients—often give plants their color and act as antioxidants, protecting them from environmental contaminants. They can do the same for you, boosting your immune system, reducing inflammation from dangerous contaminants, and fighting free-radical damage in your liver and elsewhere throughout your body.

  There are literally thousands of flavonoid compounds, so consuming a wide variety of fruits and vegetables is one way to get as many kinds as possible. Pick colorful foods such as dark beans like kidney and black beans, along with green, orange, yellow, pink, white, and red fruits and vegetables. Nuts, spices, fruit and vegetable juices (including wine), seeds, and grains also contain flavonoids.

  For specific detox support, include the following flavonoids in your daily regimen.

  ○ *Pycnogenol.* This is the brand name for a powerful antioxidant supplement made from the bark of a pine tree that grows along the coast of southwest France. It's particularly high in a class of flavonoids called oligomeric proanthocyanidins. Pycnogenol protects the liver and other gut organs from free-radical attack and helps them specifically in their detoxification role. It also aids other antioxidants in doing their job better.

- *Isotonix OPC-3.* This supplement derives its name from oligomeric proanthocyanidins (OPCs). It contains Pycnogenol as well as other good OPC sources, including bilberry, grape seed extract, red wine extracts, and citrus extract. These super antioxidants are particularly helpful in guarding the liver and the rest of your body against free-radical damage.

- *Green tea.* Enjoying a daily cup of this tasty tea is a good way to get more catechins, a particularly potent flavonoid. Black and red teas also contain catechins, but green tea has the most. Catechins offer a number of benefits, including enhancing the liver's antioxidant defenses against free radicals and protecting against liver disorders such as fatty liver disease (they block fat absorption), hepatitis, and liver cancer. As an added bonus, green tea also defends against inflammatory bowel disease as well as stomach, colorectal, esophageal, and pancreatic cancers.

- *Cocoa and dark chocolate.* Good news for chocoholics: including cocoa powder or dark chocolate in your diet helps against cirrhosis of the liver. Both are rich in flavanols, a type of flavonoid that has also been shown to promote the liver's antioxidant defenses. Incidentally, studies also show that dark chocolate and cocoa help promote healthy populations of good gut bacteria and help keep bad bacteria at bay. Of course, you won't want to indulge your chocolate cravings too much or you could gain weight. Look for chocolate products that are lower in sugar and fat.

Up next: step three of the Gut Solution—the last leg of my total wellness plan. We've seen how clearing away bad foods, habits, and substances in your life can promote better gut health and greater wellbeing. Now, we'll explore ways to bolster and strengthen your gut's natural enzymes and microflora populations so they can perform their many functions with maximum efficiency.

10

Restoring Gut Health: Supplementing with Enzymes, Probiotics, and Prebiotics

A good digestion turneth all to health.
—GEORGE HERBERT (1593–1633), "THE CHURCH-PORCH"

*U*ntil a few years ago, I thought I was pretty healthy and had no gut problems. I'd go out to one of my favorite Italian restaurants in New York, Il Mulino, and order anything I wanted—mozzarella with tomatoes, breadsticks, pasta, veal with potatoes, and a glass of wine. Sounds delicious, yes, but there was one problem. By the time I left, acid reflux had often kicked in, and I felt so bloated it was hard to keep my pants fastened.

I wondered privately what was causing all this gut turmoil. Was it the lactose in the mozzarella? Or the gluten in the breadsticks or pasta? Was it the alcohol? Still, I rarely went beyond that. I pretty much accepted feeling uncomfortable after these rich meals because I liked the food so much. I figured bloating and reflux were the price I had to pay for fine dining. I wasn't ill, but I certainly wasn't maximizing my own gut health or living as fully as I could.

Many of you probably think your gut is reasonably healthy, too. Maybe you have occasional abdominal pain or indigestion, but nothing much else of note. In other words, nothing's glaringly wrong.

But as I've said, just because you're not suffering from some diagnosed gut illness, doesn't mean you're enjoying optimum gut health either.

The truth is, if you're not practicing Gut-Smart Eating or working to Detoxify your life or to Restore your gut by taking digestive enzyme supplements, probiotics, and prebiotics, which we'll discuss in this chapter, your gut is probably not working to its fullest capacity. Your liver is likely filling up with toxins and fats and isn't cleansing your body as it should. Your intestines may be leaking so that you're only absorbing a portion of the nutrients in your food. Sure, you get enough so you don't end up with a case of rickets or scurvy or pellagra—all those vitamin-deficiency diseases we've talked about—but that doesn't mean you're getting everything you can or should get.

Someone recently said to me that most of us go through life after age thirty-five resigned to some level of bloating, fatigue, liver sluggishness, or even a mood disorder. We don't even realize that we're not feeling at the top of our game because few of us have ever really experienced the exhilaration of being truly well or the thrill of having a nontoxic, highly functioning gastrointestinal tract.

Welcome to the paradigm shift. We've begun moving from the idea of illness to the brand new world of wellness—a profound shakeup that's turning medicine upside down. Medical researchers have always been very good at defining and measuring what illness is, but not so good at pinpointing or quantifying what it actually means to be in peak health.

For years I was on board with that approach, too. I spent much of my career focused on "curing" patients who were ill. I examined a patient's heart or brain, scouring it for signs of disease, rather than thinking about optimizing its function. Likewise, if a patient didn't have rectal bleeding or extreme gastric pain right then, I assumed their gut was fine. As I began shifting my priorities to wellness, though, I realized that such old-school thinking leads to a false sense of security. Just because nothing visible is happening and you don't have obvious symptoms doesn't mean that deep down on a microscopic level there aren't changes occurring in your cells that are laying the groundwork for future problems.

And that's what medicine's new pioneers are beginning to explore. The idea is to finally define what it means to have peak health in all your organ systems, including the gut. It's not enough anymore to simply wait until someone develops GERD or an ulcer or inflammatory bowel disease or colitis. Rather, we need to pinpoint what all of us can do *right now* to preserve and enhance our gut functions—including digestion, immune defense, detoxification, and regulation of metabolism and moods (which we'll discuss in the next chapter)—so we never develop a disease.

Toward that end, new scientific questionnaires and tests are being developed to help doctors assess how well the gut is functioning—for example, how efficiently the muscles are contracting as they squeeze food through, how adept the gut is at extracting and absorbing nutrients, and how many and which kinds of intestinal bacteria are needed for optimum gut wellness. Incidentally, one of the more humorous tools (call it bathroom humor, if you will) is the Bristol Stool Scale, which divides stools into seven types, from "sausage-shaped, but lumpy" to "fluffy pieces with ragged edges" to "soft blobs with clear-cut edges." Imagine being a fly on the wall as that group of scientists sat around trying to define and categorize the motley mix of human stool shapes, textures, and colors! For a comedian, that's raw material to die for—the stuff of legendary late-night comedy skits. Seriously, though, I don't mean to poke too much fun—it's tools like these that are beginning to offer real hope to sufferers of gastrointestinal disorders who want to know what wellness looks like.

Frankly, defining gut wellness and optimizing gut function is why I wrote *No Guts, No Glory*. I want your gut to be working at the highest levels, not the minimum level. I want you to keep your gut healthy now so you don't have to focus on illness later. And if you are currently having gut problems, I want you to repair as much damage as possible and even get back to fuller or complete function as soon as possible.

My three-step Gut Solution plan is part of this new paradigm shift from illness to wellness. It's based on the latest research, and I've watched it bring both my patients and me to fuller gut health and more overall vitality. As we explore the final piece of my plan—restoring and enhancing your gastrointestinal system with supplements that work to encourage its natural functions and features—just let me say this again: I'm fully convinced by the scientific evidence and personal experience that *nobody* can achieve optimum health without focusing on the health of their gut.

SUPPLEMENTAL DIGESTIVE ENZYMES

Before we talk about enzyme supplements, I want to take you on a quick tour of your body's own enzymes at work. These astounding substances are critical participants in the digestive process and are central to keeping you alive, which is why it's so essential to support and optimize them.

Enzymes are secreted with beautifully orchestrated precision by your digestive organs to accelerate the breakdown of large macronutrients molecules (carbohydrates, proteins, and fats) so your gut can extract and distribute healthy substances, including essential micronutrients (vitamins and minerals), that are locked inside. They also assist you in absorbing these nutrients and eliminating what can't be used. Without enzymes, food would just sit in your gut and slowly rot.

There are several enzymes with specialized roles—too many to describe here—but they fall into general categories: lipases break down fats, amylases handle carbohydrates, and proteases work on proteins.

Almost as soon as you start thinking about food, enzymes begin flowing. With your first bite, amylase in your saliva starts the breakdown of complex carbohydrates into simple sugars, and salivary lipase begins digesting fats. Food travels down your esophagus to your stomach where hydrochloric acid (stomach acid)—which isn't technically a digestive enzyme but rather an enzyme helper—is secreted to activate pepsin (a protease enzyme). Together, they begin converting proteins into smaller amino acids.

Once food enters the small intestine, a round of new enzymes from the pancreas arrives. Pancreatic protease continues working on amino acids. Pancreatic amylase further converts sugar to usable glucose, and pancreatic lipase continues the breakdown of fat molecules. Lipase gets a helping hand from bile (not technically a digestive enzyme either), which emulsifies the fat so it's more easily turned into usable nutrients.

The small intestine marches out its own set of enzymes, too, to ready food molecules for absorption through its lining into the bloodstream. Interestingly, one of these is lactase, the enzyme responsible for digesting lactose in milk. You'll recall that when you're deficient in this enzyme (and about 70 percent of the world's population is) it causes lactose intolerance.

What remains of your food—the fiber—continues on to your colon for the last phase of digestion. You can't break down fiber (cellulose) yourself because you don't produce the needed enzymes called cellulases. However, your gut bacteria do produce a type of cellulase, along with other enzymes, that ferment soluble fiber (the parts of plant food that dissolve in water and become gel-like). This creates short-chain fatty acids that offer a number of health benefits. Insoluble fiber (skin, stems, and seeds from plants) remains undigested and helps form your stool, which is eventually passed out of your body as feces.

Enzyme Distress

Any of us who've had a meal and felt gaseous, bloated, and full afterward knows what it's like when something's wrong with our digestion. Of course, if we ate more slowly and consumed more nutritious, uncooked, digestible foods filled with natural enzymes, we'd have fewer gastrointestinal complaints (recall the Gut-Smart Eating Plan in Chapter 8). These include fresh, raw fruits and vegetables (including pineapple, papaya, mangos, avocados, and sprouts), along with fermented products like yogurt, non-processed cheeses, and kefir.

The beauty of consuming enzyme-rich foods is that the more you eat, the more the natural enzymes contained in them help your body's own enzymes work. You take the pressure off your enzyme supply and add to the longevity of your enzyme-producing organs. But even if you eat tons of these foods, they only contain enough enzymes to help digest themselves. Your body's enzymes still have to go it alone with other foods that may be short on enzymes from overprocessing or overcooking. And if you overeat—a problem for a lot of us—your enzymes are forced to work even harder to tackle the bigger food load. As the old proverb goes, "A man has often more trouble to digest food than to get it."

Let's face it, we live in a complex society, and one of the things that goes along with that are complex foods. I've already confessed my passion for dining out. And like everyone else, I occasionally veer off the healthy eating path. It's hard not to with so many tasty choices out there! Yes, I want everyone to eat better, but I don't want you to be so rigid that you can't enjoy an occasional dinner out or savor a burger and fries now and then. You just can't do it every day or you'll pay a price.

Sadly, that's because so much of what's in today's complex foods is nearly indigestible or outright bad for your gut. In fact, even when your digestive enzymes are flowing freely and in the right amounts, they may only be able to break down and extract about 40 to 50 percent of your food's true nutrient value. And the more refined, processed, and adulterated a food is, the lower your gut's capacity to retrieve what's there and distribute it to your body. As that old saying so wisely points out, "You can't turn straw into gold." Your digestive organs and enzymes end up working overtime, especially if you regularly eat more than you should.

The bottom line: we spend all this money on enzyme-deficient foods that are nearly impossible to digest, provide little nourishment, and wreak gut havoc. In financial terms, the return on our health investment is abysmal.

Enzyme Decline and Deficiencies

Certainly, our inability to eat well 24/7 is a very good reason to take supplemental enzymes. They help your gut's own overworked enzymes extract more of what's in your foods. But there are other compelling reasons to take them, too.

One has to do with age. As you get older, your supply of enzymes begins dwindling. It's like everything else in your body—your eyes, heart, muscles, and other organs all show diminished function with time. Studies suggest the same is true of your enzyme-making organs. In fact, by age fifty you may be making half the amount you did when you were younger. It's a double hit: not only are your enzymes working harder because of poor dietary habits, but you also have fewer of them over the years to do the work. This means you may not be digesting and absorbing all the nutrients you need as you age, and actually could be hastening the aging process.

Yet another reason to take enzyme supplements is the epidemic of enzyme deficiencies, both genetic and those created by too much stress, unhealthy foods, environmental toxins, and poor lifestyle habits. We just mentioned lactose intolerance, which begins for many people in childhood when the gene that controls lactase turns off. Of course, you may be among the lucky few with "lactase persistence," a trait that allows you to easily digest lactose throughout your life. But if you lose your ability to produce lactase—and most of us do to some degree—food containing lactose moves undigested from your small intestine to your colon where gut bacteria try to break it down unsuccessfully, resulting in cramps, diarrhea, and bloating.

Though not entirely an enzyme issue, celiac disease is nonetheless caused when digestive enzymes can't properly break down gluten (a protein found in grains like wheat and barley). This leads to an immune response that damages the small intestinal lining, contributing to leaky gut syndrome, impairing your ability to properly absorb nutrients, and causing abdominal pain and diarrhea.

There's also evidence that conditions like obesity may have an enzyme-deficiency component. For instance, some research shows that many overweight people are deficient in lipase, the fat-digesting enzyme. Without enough of it, your body stores fat, including in your arteries, leading to heart disease and other serious problems.

If you suspect you have an enzyme deficiency, talk to your doctor about getting tested. Signs of a deficiency can include gas, constipation, diarrhea, skin rashes, bloating, gastric upset, and anemia, though these are also symptoms of many other conditions. I recommend starting with Enzymedica's free online test to help pinpoint which deficiencies might be at play (see the Resources section in the back of the book).

The Toll on Your Organs

The fewer enzymes you have for whatever reason, the more it taxes your digestive organs. When your digestive organs are already damaged from bad food, stress, toxins, allergens, or medications, it spells major trouble for your gut and other organs as well as your overall health. Here's a look at what can happen:

- **Stomach.** Eating lots of junk food with few or no natural enzymes, or simply overeating, puts stress on your stomach. To help digest the overload of enzyme-deficient foods, it compensates by secreting extra stomach acid. This, in turn, can lead to or worsen acid-related conditions like ulcers and GERD. The continual pumping out of acid, which also activates more of the digestive enzyme pepsin, eventually wears out your stomach's capacity to produce both. As a result, food doesn't get properly digested and can result in everything from bloating and gas to constipation and autoimmune conditions.

- **Pancreas.** This important organ releases most of the digestive enzymes your gut uses to break down food. Substances like high-fructose corn syrup, alcohol, and medications can injure it, causing pancreatitis. With this condition, pancreatic enzymes are spurred into action before they reach the small intestine, irritating the pancreatic cells. The repercussions can be devastating. For one thing, diabetes may result if insulin-producing cells in the pancreas are harmed. Your pancreas may also be unable to send enough enzymes to your small intestine, meaning many nutrients may not be absorbed into your body to keep you healthy.

- **Liver.** We've seen how easily the liver can be damaged from too much dietary fat, alcohol, and environmental toxins. Fatty liver disease and cirrhosis are just two of the debilitating consequences. With too much damage, your liver isn't able to produce as much bile. This means fat isn't broken down properly into usable forms and neither are the fat-soluble vitamins (like A, D, and E) that it carries. Instead, fat gets stored in cells, tissues, and arteries, leading to obesity, heart disease, cancer, and other serious disorders.

- **Gallbladder.** This small organ stores bile from the liver for release in the small intestine. When bile contains too much cholesterol from a high-fat diet, gallstones may form. These hardened, pebble-like "stones" are extremely painful and may, in turn, block the flow of bile . . . and, well, you know the rest.

- **Small intestine.** Most of your body's digestion occurs here. When foods don't undergo proper breakdown because they're processed or you're not producing enough enzymes due to age or deficiencies, the larger-than-normal food particles may begin irritating the small intestinal lining, leading to leaky gut syndrome. Not only are these particles unleashed into your body through porous intestinal walls, creating autoimmune and other disorders, but the damage to your small intestine may also disrupt its ability to produce and use enzymes, creating even more enzyme dysfunction.

- **Colon.** Food that isn't fully digested ultimately moves into your
  colon. Because it's not broken down completely, the enzymes that
  your gut bacteria secrete may have a harder time digesting soluble fiber, blocking proper nutrient absorption and even leading to
  colon cancer. Insoluble fiber waste may not move out in a timely
  fashion either, resulting in constipation and other problems.

Maximizing Your Enzymes

As I've moved from being a disease doctor to a wellness doctor, I've
become more uncomfortable prescribing powerful pharmaceuticals
for digestive disorders. Few seem to cure the conditions they're aimed
at; it's as if we're covering over the problem to keep the symptoms at
bay, kind of like hanging a picture to hide a hole in the wall instead
of patching it up. And too many of these drugs cause really serious
unintended side effects. Acid suppressors like the "purple pill" and
other proton pump inhibitors, for example, significantly raise your
risk of bone fractures. It's a high price to pay—and often an unnec-
essary one—for a little reflux relief.

That's why I've gradually shifted my focus to less reliance on medicines and more reliance on gut-enhancing lifestyle changes. Indeed,
I now measure myself as a doctor not by how many medications I
give a patient, but by how many I can take away. Sure, I may need to
prescribe a drug initially for an ulcer or other condition, but the ulti-
mate goal is to shift patients away from the illness model (treating
conditions) to the wellness model (enhancing health). For me, that's
progress.

As my focus has shifted, I've also begun viewing my own gut health
differently. To handle those restaurant meals I love so much, I began
following my own advice: I cut down on unhealthy trigger foods,
worked to enhance my body's detoxification system, and started using
digestive enzyme supplements, as well as probiotics and prebiotics
(which we'll discuss in a minute).

Enzyme supplements are produced from plants, fungi, bacteria, and animal sources, and usually come in pill or powder form. You take them right before meals to heighten the action of your own digestive enzymes. (By the way, you can also take them therapeutically on an empty stomach so they're absorbed into your bloodstream to boost other systems in your body such as your cardiovascular and endocrine systems.)

I'll admit the idea of using enzymes for gut wellness was hard to get my head around at first, mainly because my training convinced me they were only for patients with serious malabsorption issues involving profound weight loss, severe diarrhea, bleeding, or vomiting. I'm talking extreme forms of digestive dysfunction like pancreatic insufficiency and bile acid disorder. I was like most physicians . . . I sympathized with patients who suffered from bloating, gaseousness, and reflux yet didn't consider them "illnesses" that needed intensive treatment—and certainly not with enzymes. Only later did I begin to understand that these symptoms are all forms of maldigestion—not a "disease" from medicine's point of view, but certainly a sign of "unwellness" that enzymes (and everything else I've been recommending) are ideally suited to address. Unfortunately, most doctors still don't "get" the benefits of enzymes and other supplements or encourage their patients to use them.

For me, the impact of supplementing with enzymes was almost immediate. Incidentally, the main culprit behind my restaurant-related reflux turned out to be a lactase deficiency triggered by the mozzarella (with a little gluten sensitivity as well). Today, before I dine, I always take a broad-spectrum enzyme supplement that helps me digest everything in my food. One of my favorites is Enzymedica's Digest Gold, along with Acid Soothe for my occasional reflux (no, I won't give up my mozzarella). These products can be purchased at almost any pharmacy or vitamin store (see the Resources section for more information). Metagenics also has an excellent line of supplements, which are available through your doctor. Now I can eat pretty much anything I want—not that I usually do or recommend it for others. Still, it's nice to know I can.

This experience has convinced me that all of us can benefit from taking digestive enzymes. In fact, when I have dinner guests over now, I hand out Digest Gold to everybody at the table!

- **Health bonuses.** Maybe you're like I was—seemingly healthy but with some hidden enzyme deficiencies that caused occasional discomfort. Or perhaps you have regular discomfort that makes mealtimes torture. Maybe you're getting older and want to preserve your own enzyme supply by giving it a helping hand, or you just want to maximize the amount of nutrients you get from your food. Whatever your situation, you should notice immediate results with supplemental enzymes.

  That's because they ease stress on your enzyme-secreting organs and help your own enzymes digest food more efficiently. They don't work on specific symptoms. They're not like antacids, for example, which suppress stomach acid but often end up making digestive problems worse (acid, after all, aids in breaking down food). With enzymes, you'll be preserving the acid status of your stomach, not trying to eliminate it! You'll have more energy and vitality, and you should also get relief from a lot of what ails your gut simply because it will be working better. Indeed, I've had patients on chronic acid medications who are living reflux- and medication-free since they started taking Digest Gold and Acid Soothe.

  Even better, with enzymes you may actually be able to *prevent* conditions like leaky gut, irritable bowel, food intolerances, and many other gut maladies. Plus, taking enzyme supplements should boost all the other functions your gut performs, including keeping your immune defenses running smoothly and communicating with your brain.

  If only I'd discovered enzyme supplements earlier—what a difference they might have made to my after-meal comfort level and my overall health. I'm just happy I have them now.

- **What to look for.** Enzyme supplements are available for nearly every need: those with a full range of enzymes to digest carbohydrates, fats, proteins, and fiber; enzymes tailored, for example, to help you just digest fats or carbohydrates; and even those for digestion of problem substances such as gluten and lactose. Refer to your results on Enzymedica's Enzyme Deficiency Test to guide you in choosing which enzyme supplements you may need to take. Here are some guidelines adapted from *Everything You Need to Know About Enzymes* (2009) by Tom Bohager to help you choose the best products:

○ *Seek enzyme supplements from reputable companies that specialize in them.* Supplement makers that manufacture many types of health products often don't have enough expertise in any single area to create the best supplements. Go with a manufacturer that specializes in digestive enzymes rather than a jack-of-all-trades.

○ *Look for a high number of active units on the label.* This is different from milligrams (mg), which is a measure of weight, not potency. The more active units, the more potential the enzymes inside have to break down different nutrients.

○ *Pay attention to pH.* All enzymes have an optimal pH and pH range in which they work best. Look on the label or in the product literature for enzyme supplements with a wide pH range (between 3 and 9). This is important because the digestive system has a wide range of pHs. For instance, the stomach averages between a pH of 2 and 3 (highly acidic), while the small intestine has a pH of 8 (very alkaline). The greater a supplement's pH range, the more likely it is to work effectively throughout the entire digestive tract.

○ *Choose products with multiple enzyme strains.* Not all lipases break down all fats. The more types of lipases included in a lipase blend, for example, the more types of fats will be digested. This blending of many enzyme strains also boosts the range of pHs in which they work.

○ *Buy no-filler formulas.* Some supplement makers use fillers, such as magnesium stearate, cellulose, pectin, maltodextrin, and talc to fill out capsules. This means you get less active ingredients per supplement, and fillers may increase the risk of an allergic reaction.

○ *Choose vegetarian capsules, not tablets.* Creating tablets can diminish the potency of enzymes, which are susceptible to heat damage. Tablets also tend to contain more fillers and binding agents.

PROBIOTIC AND PREBIOTIC SUPPLEMENTS

Recall that amazing world of beneficial microorganisms living inside your colon that we discussed in Chapters 3 and 4. Trillions of bacteria, fungi, yeast, and other microbes working together, almost like an organ, to safeguard you from toxins and harmful bacteria, assist in digestion of soluble fiber, metabolize fats, aid in the manufacture of vitamins and minerals, and communicate with your brain. They affect your moods and your immune system's disease-fighting ability and even play a role in determining how much you weigh.

When your gut environment is healthy and all the species are in proper balance, they flourish and so do you. However, when there's a disruption in their numbers or their health, bad microorganisms may begin taking over—a condition called dysbiosis that has devastating consequences for your body. In other words, your health depends on how healthy these remarkable flora and fauna helpers are. That's why, in addition to taking supplemental digestive enzymes, I believe it's crucial to also keep your gut microbial populations at optimal levels by taking probiotic supplements that contain live beneficial bacteria and prebiotic supplements that contain the food to nourish them.

Dysbiosis Devastation

So many things can upset the bacterial balance in your colon—travel, antibiotics, antacids, stress, surgery, and poor diet, to name just a few.

When dysbiosis occurs, not only is your gut affected, but the results can reach into your entire body. You may have chronic diarrhea, ongoing constipation, gas, bloating, and even bad breath. An overgrowth of candida yeast, for example, may cause a yeast infection in your rectum, or it may spill out to other organs, such as the vagina.

When things get wildly out of control it might lead to small intestinal bacterial overgrowth (SIBO). Normally, your small intestine has only a small number of microbes compared to your colon. Most are routinely swept out by muscle contractions. However, when something overturns the balance you can end up with more microbes there than you should. The result—everything from leaky gut to irritable bowel syndrome to poor nutrient absorption.

Dysbiosis is also linked to obesity. Recall the study from Chapter 4 showing that a typical American diet high in fat and sugars can promote an explosion of bacteria that extract more calories from your food and store them as fat. Not surprisingly, obese people have more of these gut microbes while thinner people carry around more bacteria that harvest fewer calories.

Scientists also believe dysbiosis may have a hand in neurological problems like ADHD, autism, depression, and anxiety conditions. That's because gut microflora play a significant part, along with your brain, in producing neurochemicals that influence your behavior and psychological well-being. When the bacterial balance is upset, especially early in life, it can interfere with proper brain development.

Also on the list of dysbiosis-related health maladies are asthma, allergies, immune system dysfunction, inflammatory bowel disease, type 1 diabetes, heart disease, and cancer. It's not hard to see why I believe it's so crucial to keep your microbial helpmates happy and functioning as they should.

Probiotics

Probiotic supplements are filled with beneficial species of active bacteria that normally populate healthy human guts. They typically come from two main species—*Lactobacillus* and *Bifidobacterium*. After taking them, these organisms remain in your colon and help keep an optimal balance of microbes.

Many foods naturally contain good bacteria, including fermented foods and beverages such as non-processed cheeses, cottage cheese, kefir, kimchi, miso, tempeh, sauerkraut, and yogurt. Some manufacturers now add extra bacteria to these and other foods during preparation, basically turning them into supplements.

Chances are your ancestors got plenty of fermented foods because before refrigeration and pasteurization it was an effective way to keep items from spoiling. Fermentation involves adding bacteria to foods that convert sugars to lactic acid. Incidentally, this is why so many fermented foods have a sour or acidic taste.

With yogurt, for example, bacteria added to milk produces lactic acid from lactose (a sugar). As the milk protein thickens and becomes acidic, it helps keep down bad bacteria that can't thrive under those conditions. When you eat yogurt and other fermented foods, the beneficial microbes contained inside not only take up residence in your gut, but the acid works its magic inside you, too, warding off unhealthy bacteria. And because fermented foods are already partially digested by the bacteria, they're easier for you to digest.

Naturally, it's a good idea to consume probiotic foods whenever you can, but since most of us don't regularly serve kimchi and kefir at meals, and because the modern world seems bent on upsetting our microbial balance at every turn, it's important to also take probiotic supplements or to consume foods fortified with beneficial microbes every day as added insurance.

It's kind of like a forest that replenishes itself with healthy new seedlings each year. The newcomers ensure a stable balance of healthy trees. In the case of probiotic supplements, you're adding in health-promoting bacteria to keep your current populations strong and vibrant and the bad bacteria in check. Incidentally, there are also new supplements on the market that combine probiotics and digestive enzymes for even more digestive benefits.

- **Health bonuses.** The scientific evidence so far on supplementing with probiotics is very impressive. They clearly help with several health conditions, including viral diarrheas, allergies, ulcerative colitis, and Crohn's disease. Researchers are also looking into using probiotics to protect against or treat everything from neurological disorders to obesity.

  Recall in Chapter 4, for instance, that rats given daily supplements of good bacteria (*Lactobacillus plantarum*) not only warded off inflammation-producing bad bacteria that promoted insulin resistance, weight gain, and type 2 diabetes, but they also remained thinner on a high-calorie diet than rats that didn't take the supplements. Rats that didn't get the probiotics and drank water containing inflammation-promoting *E. coli* bacteria put on significant weight with the same diet (Karlsson, 2011).

  Researchers are also exploring the use of probiotics (and prebiotics) to extract more health-enhancing nutrients from the foods we eat. One recent study, for example, shows that having a gut full of good bacteria helps release a potent cancer-fighting chemical called sulforaphane from broccoli (Lai, 2010).

  I have no doubt that many more studies will come along showing the profound health benefits of probiotics.

- **What to look for.** Probiotic-fortified foods and supplemental powders, capsules, and tablets are popular these days, and that's a good thing given their importance in human health. But not all of them are the same quality. It's critical to select products that have a good reputation. You obviously can't test everything yourself, but there are criteria to help you choose the highest quality products (see the Resources for manufacturers I like).

  The International Scientific Association for Probiotics and Prebiotics (ISAPP) has developed guidelines for choosing probiotics. Here are some key points to consider:

  ○ *Understand the claims.* Everything on the label should be truthful and backed by research conducted on humans and published

in reputable medical journals. Labels can state that bacteria promote health, but they can't legally tout their ability to treat, cure,
or prevent diseases. Check product websites to read study results,
and consult with your pharmacist or doctor if you need help deci-
phering the scientific findings.

◦ *Choose a reputable manufacturer.* Look for products that contain the same bacteria strains in the same amounts as the clinical
studies. Probiotics are measured in colony-forming units (CFUs),
which tell you how many live microbes per serving are in a supplement or food. They should be in the millions, or even billions.
Make sure that the number of CFUs refers to the amount of bacteria "at time of consumption," and not "at time of manufacture."
Steer clear of any product that only says "probiotic" on the label
with no mention of the types of bacteria or the CFUs. These products may not contain bacterial strains that are backed by research
or enough bacteria to bring health benefits—or they may not contain any bacteria at all.

◦ *Additional label information.* Good labels should also give you a
suggested serving size, an expiration date, proper storage instruc-
tions, and manufacturer contact information.

Prebiotics

Unlike probiotics, which introduce live bacteria into your gut, prebiotics are made mostly of carbohydrate plant fibers, called oligosaccharides, that encourage good bacteria already living inside you
to grow and thrive. Essentially, they're food for your gut microbiota,
derived from the soluble fiber that your body can't digest on its own.
Instead, your gut bacteria supply the needed enzymes to ferment
these carbohydrates. The resulting short-chain fatty acids offer many
health benefits, including feeding cells in your colon lining (and
possibly protecting them from cancer), as well as helping you
absorb essential minerals, like calcium and iron. The idea behind
consuming prebiotics is to keep populations of good bacteria in

top shape so they can perform these and other functions at an optimum level.

Prebiotic carbohydrates are found naturally in vegetables and fruits, including Jerusalem artichokes, asparagus, chicory, garlic, jicama, legumes, onions, soybeans, tomatoes, whole grains (like barley, wheat, and oats), and bananas and berries. If you eat a lot of these, your gut almost certainly contains more good microbes, and they're probably much healthier than if you subsist on a dysbiosis-promoting junk-food diet. But you really have to load up on these plant foods to gain any major prebiotic benefit.

That's why manufacturers are beginning to fortify foods, such as yogurt, nutrition bars, breads, and cereals with prebiotic fibers, and develop pills and powders that contain significantly higher amounts than what's available naturally in food.

Be on the lookout, too, for new prebiotic sources coming along. For example, goat milk was recently shown to contain high levels of prebiotic oligosaccharides, similar to that found in human milk. And European researchers believe they've discovered an important new prebiotic source—the tons of onion bulbs that are discarded each year by food manufacturers because they're too small for processing. Onions contain important prebiotic fructans.

Also new are supplements that combine prebiotics and probiotics, called synbiotics.

- **Health bonuses.** Early research on the use of prebiotics to prevent or treat dysbiosis-related diseases, such as inflammatory bowel disease and colorectal cancer, is promising. Remember that colon cells derive energy from the short-chain fatty acids produced when gut bacteria digest prebiotic carbohydrates in soluble fiber. In one new study, scientists confirmed that the colon cells of germ-free mice (raised without gut bacteria) were energy-starved and had begun digesting themselves (Donohoe, 2011). In fact, this may be what initiates the development of gastrointestinal diseases. When researchers fed the germ-free colon cells butyrate (a prebiotic carbohydrate), the animals' energy levels rose and damaging self-digestion stopped.

Researchers are also trying to create more targeted prebiotic treatments by pinpointing which carbohydrate fibers appeal most to which bacteria. This could allow them to use specific prebiotics to shift bacterial populations to desired types for health. One recent study confirmed that prebiotics are indeed effective microbe shifters (Sonnenburg, 2010). Germ-free mice were populated with two species of bacteria, one of which was particularly partial to inulin (another prebiotic carbohydrate). When inulin was added to the mice's diet, their microbial populations shifted in favor of the inulin-eating bacteria within a week or two.

- **What to look for.** As with probiotic supplements, ISAPP has also developed guidelines for choosing prebiotics. Here are some suggestions:

  ○ *Check the label.* Make sure prebiotics contain carbohydrate fibers that are known to encourage good bacteria only and not the bad kinds, too. Most prebiotics are currently designed to appeal to *Lactobacillus* and *Bifidobacterium*, but new products coming along will be tailored toward other species, too. Until they're thoroughly researched, stick with product labels that contain the following carbohydrate fibers: FOS (fructooligosaccharides), inulin, GOS (galactooligosaccharides), or TOS (transGOS). Many products say they're prebiotics, but they don't actually contain anything that encourages bacteria—beneficial or otherwise.

  ○ *Check the research.* You'll also want to see scientific evidence that prebiotic supplements and foods work in humans, and not just in animals. Only buy products that contain dosages found to be effective in the studies.

In our final chapter, we'll explore the intimate connection between the gut and the brain—a fascinating avenue of research—and what it might mean for the future of wellness medicine and your health.

11

Going with Your Gut

*I've got the guts to die. What I want to know is,
have you got the guts to live?*

—Harvey "Big Daddy" Pollitt, *Cat on a Hot Tin Roof*

*First you calculate, then you calculate again,
then you go with your gut.*

—Robert Ludlum (1927–2001), *The Sigma Protocol*

Language and literature are full of expressions involving the gut. We talk about relying on a gut feeling, listening to your gut, following your gut instincts, knowing something in your gut, having the guts to do something, spilling your guts, busting a gut, feeling gut-wrenching emotions, having a gut reaction, hating someone's guts, being gutless . . . .You get my point.

Ever wonder how and why some of these phrases came about? It's no accident, that's for sure. Most of us think of the gut in its most visible role, helping us digest our food, or as the unsavory seat of gas, cramps, and bowel movements. These top-of-mind functions have come to pretty much trump everything else. I hope that I've at least opened your eyes throughout these chapters to the gut's many other remarkable roles—from blocking pathogens through its vast immune defenses to cleansing your body of injurious substances. But I'm here to tell you the gut is even more multifaceted and amazing than that.

I've saved the best for last because it's where I think a lot of the most interesting scientific research is being done—examining the intersection between the gut and the brain. Few of us really appreciate that our guts are in intimate communication with our brains. In fact, the gut and the brain start out as a single organ during fetal development and later divide into the central nervous system (brain) and the enteric nervous system (gut). They remain connected and continue "talking" throughout our lives via a long cranial cord called the vagus nerve.

The walls of your gut actually contain millions upon millions of neurons, even more than are in your spinal cord. Not surprisingly, many scientists now think of the gut as a literal second brain. All the chemicals (including serotonin and dopamine) that circulate through your brain also swirl through your gut. Most of the functions your brain has a hand in controlling are also governed by your gut—everything from your metabolism, moods, and immune function to your weight, sleep patterns, and sex drive. In basic terms, what affects one system affects the other.

Those who first coined those expressions about the gut and wove them into our language maybe didn't understand the physiology, the anatomy, or the biology of the gut, but they must have intuitively understood something about its deep-seated and central role in our lives (yes, you might say they had a gut sense). By the way, many Eastern spiritual traditions also consider the belly or gut to be the center of profound life energy.

Perhaps science is finally catching up to what humans have always instinctively known. The gut holds a prime place of importance not only in keeping us alive but also in keeping us mentally and psychologically balanced. It's an intelligent system: sensitive, responsive, and communicative. As researchers continue unraveling the mysteries of the gut-brain connection, they're discovering ever more ways that this special alliance influences our emotional well-being and general health. They're paying closer attention, and so should you. You might even think of "going with your gut" as a fourth step in my Gut Solution plan. You've got to care for your gastrointestinal system, yes, but you also really need to put it front and center, too. Stay on intimate terms with it and trust it as a "thinking" organ. If you do, good health and vitality should follow.

TALE OF TWO BRAINS

You probably see evidence of the gut-brain connection every day and don't even realize it. Think about those butterflies in your stomach when you have to give a presentation. Or the diarrhea you get from jitters after your boss moves up a big deadline. Or even the sleeplessness that can come from trying to snooze on a full stomach. And people on antidepressants will attest to the nausea and diarrhea that often show up as side effects, just as many people with irritable bowel syndrome (IBS) know that depression and anxiety often accompany the bloating and pain. In fact, stress-reduction techniques and even low doses of antidepressants can help calm IBS symptoms.

It's clear that the gut is in constant communication with the brain and vice versa, and that they influence one another. But the implications go far beyond a twinge of nerves in your belly as you think about tomorrow's game or a case of indigestion souring your mood. In the last 100 years, scientists have found that communication dysfunctions between the brain and the gut may literally be the secret to a lot of health disorders once thought to be solely related to the brain or other organs, including autism, anxiety, obesity, and depression. Not only that, but the gut may well turn out to also be the pathway to prevention and even a cure for many of these conditions.

Let's explore how a breakdown in gut-brain signals can lead to some physical and mental afflictions.

Obesity

There are obviously many different factors involved in something as complicated as obesity, and many different theories about why people gain so much weight. But there's little doubt that communications between the gut and the brain play a role. Here's one compelling theory:

You'll recall from Chapter 5 that the stomach releases a hormone called ghrelin when it's empty. This activates a substance in your brain's hypothalamus called neuropeptide Y, which is not only involved in boosting your appetite, but also in regulating your circadian rhythms, sexual function, and responses to anxiety. After you've eaten, another hormone called leptin is secreted by your fat cells, inhibiting neuropeptide Y and letting your brain know it's time to clear away the dishes.

When everything is working well, these signals flow back and forth smoothly and reliably to keep your appetite and body weight balanced. However, when something jumbles the messages—like relentless stress—things can quickly go haywire, scrambling this beautiful feedback loop. Ghrelin and neuropeptide Y levels spike, causing cravings for high-fat, high-carb foods and helping you store them as fat more efficiently. This may have been an advantage to our ancestors during stressful times of famine when they needed to maximize calories. But because stress never seems to subside now, your gut keeps sending "eat" signals and fat continues piling up around your middle.

So where does leptin (the "I'm full" hormone) figure into all this? Interestingly, you might think obese people wouldn't have as much. However, just the opposite is true. They have higher levels of leptin. So why don't they get the signal to stop eating? It seems that obesity leads to a reduced sensitivity to leptin (leptin resistance). Therefore, even when leptin levels are high, your body doesn't sense it, and you keep eating. By the way, exercise has been shown to boost sensitivity to leptin. Yet another good reason to get up off the couch!

Add to this another piece of the obesity equation: gut bacteria. As we've seen, scientists are already starting to recognize how these organisms may have a hand in metabolism and weight gain. In fact, there's even a potential new field of science called micro-obesity that could one day help us manipulate populations of gut microbes to encourage those that make us skinny.

Sleep and Sex

In addition to stress, all these appetite-related gut-brain signals are also affected by how much you sleep. People who are sleep-deprived, possibly because of stress, secrete more ghrelin and neuropeptide Y and less leptin. Yes, that means more weight gain! Sleep deprivation and stress are also related to lower levels of sex hormones and diminished sex drive (remember, neuropeptide Y is involved in regulating both sleep and sex). Not exactly a recipe for full living, if you ask me.

Autism

We're all very distressed by the rise of this very serious neurological condition, and scientists are searching for clues about why it's on the increase. One area of active research is the gut. We've already seen that autism may be linked to having unhealthy gut bacteria, which produce substances or signals that somehow jumble brain development. One recent study also shows a possible gut-food connection. People with autism are known to have higher levels of peptides in their urine (pieces of protein that don't get broken down properly during digestion), which may circulate through the body, somehow affecting the brain (Reichelt, 2009). The source of some of these peptides is likely wheat and milk—in other words, individuals with autism may have sensitivities to gluten and casein that enters their guts in food. Though more research is needed to determine what impact these peptides actually have on the brain, the researchers noted growing evidence showing that when people with autism are put on a gluten- and casein-free diet, their peptide levels drop. Research is also beginning to show that people with autism may have a communication problem, as well, between their immune system (which you'll remember mostly resides in the gut) and their central nervous system (which is composed of the brain and spinal cord) (Goines, 2010).

Anxiety and Depression

Here's yet more evidence that gut bacteria actually talk to the brain. New research demonstrates that when genetically passive mice, raised without intestinal microorganisms, are later colonized with bacteria from assertive mice, they become more exploratory and active. Just the opposite occurs when daring, germ-free mice are populated with bacteria from more passive mice. They become less active. And, when healthy mice are given antibiotics to throw off their microbial balance, it causes a spike in brain-derived neurotrophic factor (BDNF), which plays a role in anxiety and depression (Bercik, 2011). These trillions of "outsiders" might literally be calling the shots when it comes to your behavior and well-being. All the more reason to keep them happy, so they'll keep you happy in return.

THE FUTURE OF MEDICINE

Why is the gut-brain connection so important? Why should you care? We've seen how a disruption in the signals between these two organ systems can begin a cascade of health problems that reaches into nearly every area of your life. Medicine simply hasn't been taking advantage of this special relationship. Yet the close tie between your brain and your belly might just provide the key to everything from cutting your appetite and boosting your moods to improving your sleep and even making your sex life sizzle.

Of course, the gut's potential goes way beyond just treating these particular conditions. It may turn out to be the command-and-control center for a lot of future therapies that capitalize on the gut's connection to all organ systems (not just the brain)—treatments for conditions like heart disease and cancer. That's because the gastrointestinal tract offers one of the key entryways into the body. You can't stuff things into your kidneys, but you can stuff them into your gut—beneficial things that can change the course of an illness.

I'm not just talking about pills either, which we've always relied on the gut to metabolize and distribute to areas of need inside us. No, I'm referring to new therapeutic avenues that are coming along—gut-centric treatments, tailored to work naturally with the gut, which may turn out to be far more effective than standard therapies. All the more reason to care for your gut. Chances are the more fully functional your gastrointestinal system is, the better these new treatments will work and the more you can take advantage of them. Here are a few gut-centric therapies now being explored:

- **Gut bacteria as targeted healers.** We already use probiotics (which we discussed in the last chapter) to aid in keeping our gut microflora in proper balance, helping prevent illness. We also use antibiotics to kill bad bacteria that are causing diseases (remember how they're used against *C. difficile* and *H. pylori*, the ulcer-causing germ). But I'm talking about something well beyond that—for instance, conducting DNA and RNA analyses to determine which types of bacteria, or gut types, provide which services (or damage) to the human body and how many of the good kinds are needed for optimal gut health, then using them therapeutically to treat specific disorders.

  Hippocrates, the founder of medicine, once said, "Leave your drugs in the chemist's pot if you can heal the patient with food." Of course, we're already beginning to use functional foods to feed ourselves and prebiotics to feed our gut bacteria, and it's certainly an exciting new area. But I envision actually feeding these foods to large numbers of people (and their gut microbes) as targeted "medicines" to shift bacterial populations to beneficial types and change the course of many diseases or to propel them into exquisite health, as opposed to what we're doing now: feeding people headlong into poor health and illness.

We may also unleash squads of specific bacteria known to help fight disease-causing organisms. Already we use viruses to treat cancer. We inject them into the body to carry information that alters how cells multiply. In the same way, we may employ particular types of bacteria that produce certain substances that are lethal to bad bacteria, essentially sending them into our bodies as hit men. In fact, one promising treatment for intractable *C. difficile* infections is called fecal transplant. Remember that *C. difficile* bacteria may take over a patient's gut after good bacteria are wiped out from taking antibiotics. The idea is that a donor provides feces containing a healthy blend of bacteria that's then pumped into the patient's colon to repopulate their gut and destroy the invading *C. difficile*. It's kind of like doing a "system restore" on your computer. Essentially, you're wiping out old populations of unsavory organisms and starting over with an entirely new set.

Only a handful of doctors are currently using fecal transplants, and not a lot of studies have yet looked into its effectiveness. But some researchers believe this procedure may eventually be used to treat not just *C. difficile* but many other conditions, as well, including obesity.

- **Targeted digestive enzymes and supplements.** In the future, we may routinely use various nutrients and enzymes that work in the gut to help treat specific conditions in the body and boost wellness. Several nutraceutical companies, like Enzyme Science (a new professional division of Enzymedica), Metagenics, and Horphag Research (makers of Pycnogenol), are continually looking for evidence-based data on the effectiveness of new enzyme therapies and supplements made from plant compounds, just as pharmaceutical companies are always researching chemical substances for use in medicines.

  In fact, many wellness-oriented doctors, including me, actively participate in clinical trials with these companies. For instance, one study with Enzyme Science is exploring whether an enzyme called transglucosidase, which affects starch metabolism, is effective in treating weight and metabolic syndrome. Another study is focused on supplementing with coenzyme ATP (adenosine triphosphate) to enhance our cells' ability to use energy more efficiently.

- **Altering gut function to treat gastrointestinal ailments.** Doctors may also one day rely on some of these novel therapies to treat specific gut issues that plague so many of us. For example, enzyme treatments are being developed that could help sufferers of celiac disease, assisting their gastrointestinal tracts in breaking down gluten before it reaches their small intestines and causes inflammation. Scientists are also investigating therapies that block the gluten immune response in the small intestine wall before it flares up. Right now the only effective treatment for celiac disease is to avoid gluten (which is often easier said than done since it appears in so many foods).

  Constipation—a significant issue for some 30 million Americans—may well be treated one day with a new drug currently called A3309 that takes advantage of bile acids in the gut. Recall that bile is produced by the liver to break down fats and actually works as a kind of natural laxative. Essentially, this drug-in-development blocks the small intestine from absorbing bile acids back into the bloodstream for recycling, allowing them instead to enter the colon to promote bowel movements (Wong, 2011).

- **Rethinking folk remedies for gut problems.** Yet another exciting area is the potential to use many alternative remedies that researchers are now discovering really do work. One is peppermint, which has a long history of soothing bellyaches but little scientific evidence to support its effectiveness. Now, Australian researchers have found that peppermint actually eases the pain of IBS caused from inflammation by activating an anti-pain channel in the colon called TRPM8 (Harrington, 2011). The specific pain-sensing nerve fibers that are soothed are the ones irritated by mustard and chili—a finding that makes sense since IBS sufferers often report a flare-up of symptoms after consuming spicy foods.

NO GUTS, NO GLORY

After devoting an entire book to the gut, what I'm about to say may seem a little strange. But the fact is that you can't really look at the gut in isolation. You've got to see it as part of this beautifully designed system called the human body. And in truth, your body has no walls. Every organ system communicates with every other organ system. The heart depends on the lungs and the brain. The brain depends on the gut . . . and on and on. You can't just think of taking care of your brain alone, or your joints or your eyes or your gut. They're all related and interconnected. They all impact one another.

In the future, I hope to highlight some of these other organ systems and their role in your overall health so we'll be able to put it all together and live with a bigger picture in mind. But we can only explore one system at a time. We're spotlighting the gut here because of its crucial link to your brain and to every other organ system via nerve endings, blood vessels, and hormones. By now, you should appreciate that if you maltreat your gut, the ramifications—the collateral damage—will be felt in your knee or your brain or your heart . . . or even in your bedroom! Its remarkable reach in the human body, from head to toe, is truly breathtaking, and scientists will no doubt continue discovering new things about it all the time.

No Guts, No Glory is really about going with your gut instead of ignoring or abusing it, putting it first, and heeding its desire to be nurtured in the ways it was designed for. It's about listening to your gut, hearing its messages that signal something's wrong. If you let it, your gut can offer abundant clues to what ails you. It's also about celebrating if all you hear is silence—the lovely silence of a well-oiled machine. It's about losing habits that undermine gut health and taking steps to maximize its function so all your other organ systems—and you—function better.

For me, the phrase "no guts, no glory" really sums up my message. Yes, it usually refers to war or sports; the idea being that if you don't have courage—if you don't give the battle or game your all—you won't ever know the sweet smell of victory. But the same can be said of your gut. If you don't give it your all—if you don't keep it in fighting shape—you won't ever know the sweet smell of vitality and health. This is the path to true wellness, more energy, greater well-being, and a richer life. It's the secret I promised to share with you back in the first chapter—a secret I hope you'll now share with others. And it's also my guarantee. Follow my three-part Gut Solution plan, make it the core of your total wellness regimen, and full health and vibrancy can be yours, too. All it takes is guts.

Resources

ADDICTION AND TREATMENT

GreenFacts
Website: www.greenfacts.org/en/
psychoactive-drugs/index.htm
Information on psychoactive drugs, alcohol, tobacco, and illicit substances, as well as approaches and resources for breaking addictions

National Institute on Drug Abuse
Website: http://www.nida.nih.gov/
nidahome.html
Information on the science of drug abuse and addiction

DETOXIFICATION

Metagenics
100 Avenida La Pata
San Clemente, CA 92673
Phone: 800-692-9400
Website: www.metagenics.com
Makers of GlutaClear and developers

of the ClearPath detoxification and healthy lifestyle program, available through licensed health care providers

Ortho Molecular Products
1991 Duncan Place
Woodstock, IL 60098
Phone: 800-332-2351
Website: www.orthomolecular
products.com
Developers of the Core Restore BT detoxification and healthy lifestyle program, available through health care professionals

DIGESTIVE ENZYME FORMULAS

Enzymedica, Inc.
752 Tamiami Trail
Port Charlotte, FL 33953
Phone: 888-918-1118
Website: www.enzymedica.com
Makers of Digest Gold, Acid Soothe, and other enzyme supplements

Enzyme Science
750 Tamiami Trail
Port Charlotte, FL 33953
Phone: 855-281-7246
Website: www.enzyscience.com
Available only through health care professionals. Enzyme Science is a professional division of Enzymedica

Genesis Today, Inc.
14101 West Highway 290
Building 1900
Austin, TX 78737
Phone: 800-916-6642
Website: www.genesistoday.com

Market America
Phone: 866-420-1709
Website: www.marketamerica.com/index.cfm
Makers of Isotonix and other enzyme supplement brands

Metagenics
100 Avenida La Pata
San Clemente, CA 92673
Phone: 800-692-9400
Website: www.metagenics.com
Makers of SpectraZyme and Metazyme, as well as other types of gastrointestinal dietary aids, available through licensed health care providers

Ortho Molecular Products
1991 Duncan Place
Woodstock, IL 60098
Phone: 800-332-2351

Website: www.orthomolecular products.com
Available through health care professionals

ELIMINATION DIET

Institute for Functional Medicine
Website: www.functionalmedicine.org/content_management/files/ifm_Comp_Elim_Diet_091503.pdf
Guidelines for a seven-day elimination diet

WebMD
Website: www.webmd.com/allergies/allergies-elimination-diet
Elimination diet and food challenge test for diagnosing allergies

ENVIRONMENTAL TOXINS (INFORMATION)

American Lung Association
Website: www.stateoftheair.org/2011/assets/SOTA2011.pdf
State of the Air 2011 Report

Centers for Disease Control and Prevention
Website: www.cdc.gov/exposure report
National Report on Human Exposure to Environmental Chemicals (2011)

Environmental Working Group

Website: www.ewg.org/tap-water/home
National database of pollutants in tap water (2009)

Website: www.ewg.org/featured/15
Research documenting the health effects of environmental toxins in the body from grandparents to babies (2011)

ENZYME DEFICIENCY TEST

Enzymedica
Website: www.Enzymedica.com/takethetest
Free online test to help pinpoint enzyme deficiencies

FARMERS' MARKETS AND COMMUNITY-SPONSORED AGRICULTURE (CSA)

Local Harvest
PO Box 1292
Santa Cruz, CA 95061
Phone: 831-515-5602
Website: www.localharvest.org
Source for farmers' markets and CSA farms that offer organic, locally grown produce and meats near you

FASTING

WebMD
Website: www.webmd.com/diet/fasting
Overview of fasting diets

FUNCTIONAL/MEDICAL FOODS

Deplin
Website: www.deplin.com
Makers of Deplin, a medical food treatment for depression, available through health care professionals

LifeMax, Inc.
7576 Kingspointe Parkway, Suite 160
Orlando, FL 32819
Phone: 407-248-8499
Website: http://home.lifemax.net or http://theperfectgrain.com
Makers of Mila

Metagenics
100 Avenida La Pata
San Clemente, CA 92673
Phone: 800-692-9400
Website: www.metagenics.com
Makers of UltraMeal Plus 360 and UltraInflamX Plus 360, as well as and other gastrointestinal dietary aids, available through licensed health care professionals

GLYCEMIC INDEX

Glycemic Index Foundation
Website: www.glycemicindex.com
Glycemic index and database

LACTOSE INTOLERANCE

Lactaid
Website: www.lactaid.com
Phone: 800-522-8243 or
    800-LACTAID
Products and supplements for people with lactose intolerance

NUTRITION INFORMATION

McKinley Health Center
Website: www.mckinley.illinois.edu
    /handouts/macronutrients.htm
Information on what each macro-nutrient does and foods that contain them

Nutrition.gov
Website: www.nutrition.gov/nal_
    display/index.php?info_center=
    11&tax_level=2&tax_subject=
    388&topic_id=1668&placement
    _default=0
Databases of antioxidant and phyto-nutrient content of foods

NutritionMD
Website: www.nutritionmd.org/
    index.html
Source for comprehensive nutrition information operated by Physicians Committee for Responsible Medicine

Website: www.nutritionmd.org/
    health_care_providers/general_
    nutrition/micro_table2.html
List of essential vitamins, their roles, and Recommended Dietary Allowances (RDAs) by age

Website: www.nutritionmd.org/
    health_care_providers/general_
    nutrition/micro_table3.html
List of essential minerals, their roles, and RDAs by age

Website: www.nutritionmd.org/
    health_care_providers/general_
    nutrition/lifetime_nutrition_
    requirements.html
Nutritional requirements throughout the life cycle from adolescence to adulthood

Metagenics
Website: www.metagenics.com/
    patients/learning-center/
    nutrition-101
Basic guidelines for eating a healthy diet

RawFoodExplained.com
Website: www.rawfoodexplained
    .com/the-physiology-of-
    digestion/the-physiological-
    determinants-of-the-optimum-
    diet.html
Description of the physiological features that helped determine the optimum diet for humans

U.S. Department of Agriculture
Website: www.nal.usda.gov/fnic/
foodcomp/Data/HG72/hg72_
2002.pdf
*Information on estimating portion
sizes, daily dietary intakes of
nutrients, food sources of nutrients,
and nutritive value of specific foods*

ISOTONIX OPC-3 SUPPLEMENTS

Market America
Phone: 866-420-1709
Website: www.marketamerica
.com/index.cfm
*Makers of Isotonix and other
supplement brands*

PROBIOTIC AND PREBIOTIC FORMULAS

Enzymedica, Inc.
752 Tamiami Trail
Port Charlotte, FL 33953
Phone: 888-918-1118
Website: www.enzymedica.com

Enzyme Science
750 Tamiami Trail
Port Charlotte, FL 33953
Phone: 855-281-7246
Website: www.enzyscience.com/
*Available only through health care
professionals; Enzyme Science is a
professional division of Enzymedica*

Metagenics
100 Avenida La Pata
San Clemente, CA 92673
Phone: 800-692-9400
Website: www.metagenics.com
*Available through licensed health
care professionals*

Market America
Phone: 866-420-1709
Website: www.marketamerica
.com/index.cfm
*Makers of Isotonix and other
supplement brands*

Ortho Molecular Products
1991 Duncan Place
Woodstock, IL 60098
Phone: 800-332-2351
Website: www.orthomolecular
products.com
*Available through health care
professionals*

PYCNOGENOL SUPPLEMENTS

**Horphag Research Ltd./
Natural Health Science Inc.**
5 Marine View Plaza, Suite 403
Hoboken, NJ 07030
Phone: 877-369-9934
Website: www.pycnogenol.com

Market America
Phone: 866-420-1709
Website: www.marketamerica
   .com/index.cfm
*Makers of Isotonix OPC-3 with
Pycnogenol*

RELAXATION AND SLEEP

HelpGuide.org
Website: http://helpguide.org/
   mental/stress_management_
   relief_coping.htm
*Suggestions for preventing, reducing,
and coping with stress*

WebMD
Website: www.webmd.com/sleep-
   disorders/guide/sleep-hygiene
*Sleep hygiene solutions for getting a
better sleep*

Bibliography

American Lung Association. "State of the Air Report, 2011." Available online at: www.stateoftheair.org/2011/assets/SOTA2011.pdf.

Bailey, Michael T., Scott E. Dowd, Jeffrey D. Galley, et al. "Exposure to a Social Stressor Alters the Structure of the Intestinal Microbiota: Implications for Stressor-Induced Immunomodulation." *Brain, Behavior, and Immunity*, 2011; 25 (3): 397–407.

Barrett, Julie R., "Chemical Exposures: The Ugly Side of Beauty Products." *Environmental Health Perspectives*, 2005; 113 (1): A24.

Bercik, Premysl, Emmanuel Denou, Josh Collins, et al. "The Intestinal Microbiota Affect Central Levels of Brain-Derived Neurotropic Factor and Behavior in Mice." *Gastroenterology*, 2011; 141 (2): 599–609.

Bohager, Tom. *Everything You Need to Know about Enzymes*. Austin, TX: Greenleaf Book Group Press, 2009.

Carone, Benjamin R., Lucas Fauquier, Naomi Habib, et al. "Paternally Induced Transgenerational Environmental Reprogramming of Metabolic Gene Expression in Mammals." *Cell*, 2010; 143 (7): 1084–1096.

Centers for Disease Control and Prevention. "National Report on Human Exposure to Environmental Chemicals" (June 2011). Available online at: www.cdc.gov/exposurereport.

Donohoe, Dallas R., Nikhil Garge, Xinxin Zhang, et al. "The Microbiome and Butyrate Regulate Energy Metabolism and Autophagy in the Mammalian Colon." *Cell Metabolism*, 2011; 13 (5): 517–526.

Environmental Working Group. "National Drinking Water Database" (Dec 2009). Available online at: www.ewg.org/tap-water/home.

Environmental Working Group. "The Environment: BodyBurden" (2011). Available online at: www.ewg.org/featured/15.

Gershon, Michael. *The Second Brain.* New York, NY: HarperCollins, 1998.

Goines, Paula and Judy Van de Water. "The Immune System's Role in the Biology of Autism." *Current Opinion in Neurology,* 2010; 23 (2): 111–117.

Hammons, Amber J. and Barbara H. Fiese. "Is Frequency of Shared Family Meals Related to the Nutritional Health of Children and Adolescents?" *Pediatrics.* 2011; 127 (6): e1565–e1574.

Harrington, Andrea M., Patrick A. Hughes, Christopher M. Martin, et al. "A Novel Role for TRPM8 in Visceral Afferent Function." *Pain,* 2011; 152 (7): 1459–1468.

Howard, Amber L., Monique Robinson, Grant J. Smith, et al. "ADHD Is Associated with a 'Western' Dietary Pattern in Adolescents." *Journal of Attention Disorders,* 2011; 15 (5): 403–411.

Inafuku, Masashi, Koji Nagao, Saori Nomura, et al. "Protective Effects of Fractional Extracts from *Panellus serotinus* on Non-alcoholic Fatty Liver Disease in Obese, Diabetic db/db Mice." *British Journal of Nutrition,* 2011 July 26: 1–8.

International Food Information Council Foundation. "Background on Functional Foods" (August 2011). Available online at: www.foodinsight.org/Resources/Detail.aspx?topic=Background_on_Functional_Foods.

International Scientific Association for Probiotics and Prebiotics. "Probiotics: A Consumer Guide for Making Smart Choices" (March 2009); available online at: www.isapp.net/docs/Consumer_Guidelines-probiotic.pdf. Also, "Prebiotics: A Consumer Guide for Making Smart Choices" (March 2009); available online at: www.isapp.net/docs/Consumer_Guidelines-prebiotic.pdf.

Kaddurah-Daouk, Rima, Rebecca A. Baillie, Hongjie Zhu, et al. "Enteric Microbiome Metabolites Correlate with Response to Simvastatin Treatment." PLoS ONE, 2011; 6 (10): e25482.

Karlsson, Caroline L.J., Göran Molin, Frida Fåk, et al. "Effects on Weight Gain and Gut Microbiota in Rats Given Bacterial Supplements and a High-Energy-Dense Diet from Fetal Life Through to 6 Months of Age." *British Journal of Nutrition,* 2011; 106 (6): 887–895.

Kurppa, Kalle and Katri Kaukinen. "Should Screen-Detected and Asymptomatic Celiac Patients Be Treated? A Prospective and Randomized Trial." *Digestive Disease Week*, 2011: Abstract 620; presented May 9, 2011.

Lai, Ren-Hau, Miller, Michael J., Jeffery, Elizabeth. "Glucoraphanin Hydrolysis by Microbiota in the Rat Cecum Results in Sulforaphane Absorption." *Food & Function*, 2010; 1 (2): 161–166.

Ley, Ruth E., Peter J. Turnbaugh, Samuel Klein, et al. "Microbial Ecology: Human Gut Microbes Associated with Obesity." *Nature*, 2006; 444 (7122): 1022–1023.

Martin, François-Pierre J., Marc-Emmanuel Dumas, Yulan Wang, et al. "A Top-Down Systems Biology View of Microbiome-Mammalian Metabolic Interactions in a Mouse Model." *Journal of Molecular Systems Biology;* 3 (112), published online May 22, 2007. doi:10.1038/msb4100153.

Mozaffarian, Dariush, Tao Hao, Eric B. Rimm, et al. "Changes in Diet and Lifestyle and Long-Term Weight Gain in Women and Men." *New England Journal of Medicine*, 2011; 364 (25): 2392–2404.

Nagao, Koji, Nao Inouea, Masashi Inafuku, et al. "Mukitake Mushroom (*Panellus serotinus*) Alleviates Nonalcoholic Fatty Liver Disease Through the Suppression of Monocyte Chemoattractant Protein 1 Production in db/db Mice." *Journal of Nutritional Biochemistry*, 2010; 21 (5): 418–423.

National Digestive Diseases Information Clearinghouse. "Your Digestive System and How It Works" (Apr 2008). Available online at: http://digestive.niddk.nih.gov/ddiseases/pubs/yrdd.

Parracho, H. M., M.O. Bingham, G.R. Gibson, et al. (2005). "Differences Between the Gut Microflora of Children with Autistic Spectrum Disorders and That of Healthy Children." *Journal of Medicinal Microbiology*, 2005; 54 (10): 987–991.

RawFoodExplained.com. "The Physiological Determinants of the Optimum Diet." Available online at: www.rawfoodexplained.com/the-physiology-of-digestion/the-physiological-determinants-of-the-optimum-diet.html.

Reichelt, K.L. and A.M. Knivsberg. "The Possibility and Probability of a Gut-to-Brain Connection in Autism." *Annals of Clinical Psychiatry* 2009; 21 (4): 205–211.

Sonnenburg, Erica D., Hongjun Zheng, Payal Joglekar, et al. "Specificity of Polysaccharide Use in Intestinal Bacteroides Species Determines Diet-Induced Microbiota Alterations." *Cell*, 2010; 141 (7): 1241–1252.

SustainableTable.com. "Food Additives Pose Threat." Available online at: www.sustainabletable.org/issues/additives.

Van Oudenhove, Lukas, Shane McKie, Daniel Lassman, et al. "Fatty Acid-Induced Gut-Brain Signaling Attenuates Neural and Behavioral Effects of Sad Emotion in Humans." *Journal of Clinical Investigation*, 2011; 121 (8), 3094–3099.

Wang, Zeneng, Elizabeth Klipfell, Brian J. Bennett, et al. "Gut Flora Metabolism of Phosphatidylcholine Promotes Cardiovascular Disease." *Nature*, 2011; 472 (7341): 57–63.

Wong, Banny S., Michael Camilleri, Sanna McKinzie, et al. "Effects of A3309, an Ileal Bile Acid Transporter Inhibitor, on Colonic Transit and Symptoms in Females with Functional Constipation." *American Journal of Gastroenterology*, 2011 August 30; doi:10.1038/ajg.2011.285.

Index

About the Authors

Steven Lamm, M.D.

Steven Lamm appears regularly as the "house doctor" on the ABC program *The View*. He also offers twice-weekly health advice on LXNY, seen throughout the New York-New Jersey metropolitan area. He has been a frequent commentator on *The Today Show*, as well as having been a guest on *Oprah*, *Nightline*, and *Late Night with Conan O'Brien*. He is known for his authoritative, entertaining, and always current information.

No Guts, No Glory is Dr. Lamm's fifth book, and as with his previous books, *Thinner at Last* and *The Virility Solution*, he continues challenging the reader to achieve new levels of health and vitality. His last book, *The Hardness Factor*, communicated the idea that sexual function is linked to cardiovascular health.

Dr. Lamm is an internist on the faculty of New York University, and has taught students and residents for thirty years. He has an internal medicine practice in New York City, and is daily promoting the idea that the absence of illness does not mean you are well.

Sidney Stevens

Sidney Stevens is a veteran writer and journalist. In addition to collaborating on several health books, her writing has also appeared in *Newsweek, Consumer Reports Money Adviser, Sierra, Mother Nature Network, Travel & Leisure, Real Woman,* and other publications. Visit her website at www.sidneystevens.com.

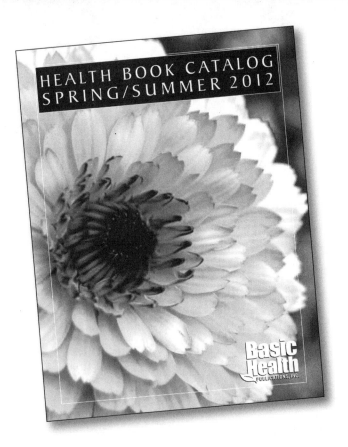